with Older People

Best Practice with Older People

Social Work Stories

KAREN JONES
AND
SUSANNA WATSON

palgrave
macmillan

First published 2013 by
PALGRAVE MACMILLAN

Palgrave Macmillan in the UK is an imprint of Macmillan Publishers Limited, registered in England, company number 785998, of Houndmills, Basingstoke, Hampshire RG21 6XS.

Palgrave Macmillan in the US is a division of St Martin's Press LLC, 175 Fifth Avenue, New York, NY 10010.

Palgrave Macmillan is the global academic imprint of the above companies and has companies and representatives throughout the world.

Palgrave® and Macmillan® are registered trademarks in the United States, the United Kingdom, Europe and other countries

ISBN: 978–0–230–29382–3

This book is printed on paper suitable for recycling and made from fully managed and sustained forest sources. Logging, pulping and manufacturing processes are expected to conform to the environmental regulations of the country of origin.

A catalogue record for this book is available from the British Library.

A catalog record for this book is available from the Library of Congress.

This book is dedicated to the 12 social workers who shared their stories with us and to the many others whose daily work with older people is equally compassionate, intelligent and insightful.

Contents

1 Introduction

This is a book which places the actual practice of social work with older people firmly centre stage. At its heart are 12 accounts of social work as told by social workers themselves, in which they describe what happened, the relationships they built, the knowledge they used, how they felt and the decisions they made. The stories are rich in detail and each is used to illustrate, examine and discuss what social work looks like when it is done well. If you are new to social work with older people, you will be given a good idea of what the work really entails and the ways in which social workers approach the situations in which they and their clients find themselves. You can start to think for yourself about what you would have done and why. If you are an experienced social worker, we hope you will recognise your own work in what you read and that this will help you to analyse, critique and celebrate what you do.

Each story involves at least one older person. However, whilst age is a common thread running through all the accounts, each one also concerns a unique individual or group of individuals with their own particular needs and strengths. Some of the situations described involve life changes or crises associated with ageing, but many others have their origins in long-standing health or relationship issues that happen to be explored here within a context of older age. So, many of the stories and much of the analysis that accompanies them is equally relevant to social work with adults of any age.

In the chapters that follow, we take an unashamedly positive approach, looking for the 'best' in the work we were told about. We are, in a sense, acting as advocates for the profession and sharing our belief that there is very good work going on much of the time, which is often unacknowledged. In doing so, we are not denying that social work is in need of reform or that the context in which we work is deeply flawed. Nor are we claiming that the practice we describe is any sense perfect. In fact, as we shall see, social work is at its best when it adopts a critical and self-questioning stance – one that understands that there is very rarely an objectively 'best' course of action. (What is best for a woman with dementia may not be best for the daughter who is struggling to care for her. What is best in the judgement of the social worker may not be wanted by the client.) However, what we are trying to do is to show how social workers go about answering the question posed by David Howe: 'What is the best course of action in this case?' (Howe, 2009, p. 201). Howe argues that answering this question is essentially a matter of judgement based on an analysis of factual information, subjective opinions, theoretical frameworks, research, critical thinking and ethical reasoning.

Any judgement will (and should) be open to debate. With this in mind, we have not written the sort of book that attempts to provide a blueprint for practice. Many other text books address the question of 'how to do' social work with older people far more explicitly. Instead, we take a 'bottom-up' approach, in the tradition of narrative and reflective writing, using stories of day-to-day social work as a way of raising questions and engaging the reader in a debate about what good practice looks like. While we draw out a number of strong and often recurring topics and ideas, we have avoided an explicitly thematic approach. This means that you will not find a chapter on this skill or that methodology. Instead, what is distinctive about the 'best practice' approach taken here is that it starts with real practice done well and draws out learning from that practice. In this respect it has much in common with the way pre-qualifying students and social workers completing Continuing Professional Development (CPD) portfolios are expected to analyse the work they do with their clients. We hope that by integrating an exploration of knowledge, skills and values with actual practice, we have therefore provided a helpful model for both students and experienced practitioners.

The shape of the book

The stories we tell in the following chapters are taken from interviews with a number of social workers employed by different local authorities. In each case, we asked them to describe some practice about which they felt positive. Once they had started talking, they all spoke enthusiastically (and at length) with very little prompting, although sometimes we asked questions to clarify specific points. It should go without saying that this book is not claiming to be research.

The social workers chose what they wanted to talk about, so the work described here does not reflect every aspect of social work with older people. While much of it involves considerable complexity, the social workers were unlikely to talk about clients with whom they had not been able to form good relationships or situations where they felt too ambivalent about the outcome to see it as obviously positive. They were also unlikely to select cases which were routine and not overtly challenging. For this reason, straightforward assessments and brief interventions, where the principal requirements are an ability to listen and give sound information and advice, are under-represented here. The stories are told from the social workers' point of view and other people, including their clients, may well have experienced it very differently. As writers, we have also shaped what was said, highlighting what seemed to us to be important. Simply by creating a beginning and an end to the stories, we have given a narrative shape to something that was often, in reality, more like an excerpt from an ongoing and changing situation. As one of the social workers said, unsure where to end her interview:

> People's lives just shift and change and move on – it's [a question of] where you want to place that full stop.

So, the cases were picked by the social workers because they felt that they had been able to get involved and create an impact, not because they were representative of their case loads as a whole. At the same time, our experience as a teacher and a practitioner suggests that they are not wholly exceptional. Although social work with older people is often characterised as short-term and rather routine (Hugman, 2000), the reality is that many cases are complex and offer plenty of scope for social workers to use their skills (a topic we will return to in Chapter 6). Most social workers will have several of these complex cases on their case load, which are likely to take up a disproportionate amount of their time. So we would maintain that most of the social work we have written about is very much a part of the practice that makes up the life of front-line social workers. It is not practice that is either idealised or unattainable.

The book is divided into four broadly themed sections, each of which has an opening chapter followed by three case studies. The chapters at the start of each section give a brief context to the theme and draw together some of the characteristics of good social work embodied in the case studies. They provide both an analysis of the relationship between social work theory and the practice that follows and an overview of the 'legal and procedural realities' (Jones et al., 2008b, p. 287) in which that practice takes place.

Each case study chapter begins with three 'questions to ask yourself as you read'. We hope that these will provide a useful way into thinking about the content, although additional questions, issues and points for debate will certainly occur to individual readers. The case studies are based on a single interview. The 'story' is told first, with very little comment, in order to encourage readers to respond themselves before reading our response in the discussion at the end. We hope that this will be a useful format for teaching and learning, as the story can easily be extracted and used to stimulate debate. At the same time, we would encourage as many readers as possible to start at the beginning and read the book as a whole. Much of its power is in the cumulative effect of the 12 stories, which together say a great deal about what is best and why in social work with older people.

Part of what we are trying to capture is the authentic detail of the work, so we were very conscious of the potential difficulties in relation to confidentiality. Even though what we were doing was not 'research', we did gain approval from a university ethics committee as well as the agreement of directors of the social services departments involved. The social workers we spoke to were given the opportunity to read a draft of the chapter that was based on their interview and raise any concerns at that stage. And, of course, the names of the social workers, their clients and much biographical detail has been changed or made up to protect their anonymity.

The importance of the 'best practice' approach

Before moving on to the practice examples themselves, we want to spend some time looking at the importance of the 'best practice approach' to social work analysis.

The concept was originally put forward as 'critical best practice' in an article by Harry Ferguson in the *British Journal of Social Work* (2003) and, since then, has been developed in an edited collection, *Best Practice in Social Work: Critical Perspectives* (Jones et al., 2008a), and in the book by David Howe (2009), which we referred to earlier. Examples of practice in social work books frequently take the form of brief case studies, created to illustrate a particular point. By contrast, the best practice approach is a way of thinking and writing about social work which takes as its starting point a detailed description of practice and uses this as a way of interpreting practice and facilitating learning from it. It is a simple idea, but is perhaps unique in its emphasis on capturing in detail 'the very "work" that is social work, the actions taken, what gets said and done and with what consequences' (Ferguson, 2008, p. 17). We believe that this approach to analysing social work is important in a number of ways, which are discussed in some detail below.

Creating a dialogue between theory and practice

The theory base of social work is complex and sometimes contradictory, drawing as it does on many different academic disciplines and schools of thought. David Howe (2009) suggests that this abundance is inevitable in a profession that deals with individuals and society, arguing that the many ways of thinking about our work should serve to keep us engaged and fascinated by what we do. However, while social workers may be inspired, intrigued and excited, it can also be challenging to realise that individual theories or methods cannot by themselves offer a comprehensive blueprint for practice. For example, social workers might use their understanding of task-centred approaches to work with a service user in a pragmatic, problem-solving way. When working with older people however, it is unlikely that this would exemplify 'task-centred theory' in its purest form. Realistically, there often would not be time, in addition to which, many of the situations social workers are involved in are simply too complex, ambiguous and changing for this to be possible. Similarly, however committed social workers may be to the broad principles of 'anti-oppressive practice', they often struggle to analyse the detail of their work within an anti-oppressive framework. As Wilson and Beresford (2000) point out, from a service user perspective it is highly questionable whether statutory social workers can ever really claim that anti-oppressive practice defines what they do.

Even research and 'evidence-based practice' can seem remote from day to day social work. Sheldon and Macdonald (2009) suggest that much of the research relevant to social work is around the effectiveness of particular types of service (homecare, telecare, rehabilitation). This is important for service development, but remains one step removed from actual social work practice. They also highlight research suggesting that care arrangements are more effective when social workers are able to take time to build a relationship with their clients. This is an important finding, which social workers might use to convince their agencies that it is counterproductive for them to work as quickly and superficially as they are sometimes asked to do. However, it would still not really help them to decide what to do in a particular circumstance with a particular client (quite apart from the fact that the conclusion seems too obvious to have warranted the research in the first place).

So, while theories, methods and research are crucial in helping social workers to understand the people and situations they encounter, they do not define the practice itself. In fact, there is an important sense in which social work does not even exist 'in theory'. It can only be practised, which means it is inevitably influenced, changed and constrained by the social, political and cultural world in which it finds itself. This does not mean, however, that social work practice has no identity of its own and cannot be theorised. Social workers need to have an understanding of how people develop, think and feel and how society is organised and we need to be able to articulate what we are doing, and why, in the light of that understanding.

Perhaps the problem lies not so much in the theories themselves but in the way in which their relationship to social work practice is understood. This is not a new conundrum. In the very first year of the *British Journal of Social Work*, Olive Stevenson was arguing that theories should be understood as 'frames of reference' – ways of thinking about and organising what we do, not as ideas that define practice. Theories help people to identify patterns from a distance, find connections and establish a general view. From a distance 'the common elements in people's appearance may dominate the eye' (Stevenson, 1971, p. 229) and you can see the shape of the whole. However, as you get closer to the individual, as social workers do, you start to see the detail and the differences. Deciding what to do becomes a question less of theory than of informed judgement.

More recently, there has been a growing interest in bringing social work theory and practice closer together, so that writing about social work increasingly acknowledges the complexity and uncertainty of what is involved in doing it. And yet, there remains a tendency to see theory as something that has to be 'applied' to practice – or to which, practice must be made to fit. This book, jointly written by a social work academic and a social work practitioner, is aiming to do something very different. In drawing out the detail of practice itself, the best practice approach seeks to test, refine and critique the more abstract ideas about social work, creating a dialogue between theory and practice. Social workers need, for example, to have read and thought about the ways in which power is exercised in a 'helping relationship'. But, what does this mean sitting in front of Mrs Smith at this particular time on this particular day with this particular decision that needs to be made? When this work with this person is looked at in detail, how does it change, fine-tune, confirm or undermine our theoretical understanding?

Tackling the deficit

This lack of clarity about the relationship between social work theory and practice has contributed much to social work's overall lack of confidence in itself. Despite the work within social work education and training to bring theory and practice closer together, much of the writing about social work in academic journals is based on quasi-scientific research, communicated in fairly impenetrable language. This may give the discipline 'an aura of authority' in university circles (Witkin, 2000, p. 389) and attract funding to university departments, but it also serves to alienate the vast majority of social work practitioners. At the opposite extreme, some text book accounts focus on the wholly pragmatic, suggesting that social work is an activity which can be mastered with the right 'competencies'. This, coupled with the managerialism of most social services departments, creates a dangerously reductionist view of good practice as a matter primarily of technical proficiency. While such an approach may superficially remove practitioners' (and their agencies') sense of uncertainty about what they are doing, it is ultimately an anxious and defensive position. Far from building real confidence, it acts (along with the processes, procedures and forms that accompany it) as a kind of professional armour against the relationship-building, reflection, self-questioning and critical thinking that good social work requires.

Academic writing has also tended to focus on what could be done better, on the not-quite-good-enough. This leads Ferguson to conclude that social work has been left

> without a knowledge base of critical best practice and devoid of a tradition of celebration, pride or sense of achievement on which to build or fall back and has helped to create a context where governments can feel able to ride roughshod over social work. (Ferguson, 2003, p. 1008)

In fact, the last ten years have seen several developments in social work theory, ideas and research which do seek to promote a more explicitly positive approach, including constructive and strengths-based practice methods and narrative and service user led approaches to research. We would argue, however, that there are still gaps in the literature relating to

7

the ways in which good practice can itself be theorised and showcased, rather than simply aspired to. In our experience of practice and teaching, many social workers themselves have internalised a kind of negativity. They are often reticent about what they see as 'blowing their own trumpets', finding it easier to talk about what has not been achieved because of lack of resources, the unfairness of society or the absence of an obviously successful outcome. There is a nostalgia for the 'good old days' of casework and an assumption that, since the advent of care management, social work (particularly with older people) has lost its soul and been reduced to the 'low level functional tasks' (Webb, 2006, p. 73). It is certainly true that the managerial transformation of social work has done a lot of damage but, as the following chapters show, characterising social work as a series of 'functional tasks' is very far from the whole truth. At the same time, if it is repeated often enough, social workers will start to believe it and, once they believe it, they are more likely to think about (and go about) their own practice in a limited and limiting way.

It is this atmosphere of anxious negativity, along with persistent criticism from the media, politicians and the public, that Ferguson (2003) refers to as social work's 'deficit culture' – something the best practice approach is explicitly trying to counteract. It is a culture that was recognised by the Social Work Task Force (set up after the death of 'Baby P' to begin the process of social work reform), when they called for

> a continuously refreshed 'bank' of stories and case studies that help to illustrate good social work practice, creating a benchmark for the public of the positive impact social workers can have. (Social Work Task Force, 2009, p. 49)

This book does that in an obvious way and we hope that our 12 case studies will go some way towards refreshing the bank. But, with the best practice approach, we are not just illustrating practice, we are also opening up a dialogue about what good social work is like. This is a conversation in which confident and self-aware practitioners everywhere can participate.

Process as well as outcome

One of the difficulties for social workers, especially in an age where everything is judged by its 'outcome', is that the result of their intervention is often not obviously 'good'. In many situations (though by no means all, as the work described in the following chapters will testify), the best that can be achieved is to prevent someone's circumstances getting worse or to make them slightly more manageable. One of the social workers we spoke to told us about a woman she had worked with who was a chronic alcoholic and was being exploited by members of her family, who took her money and used her house to drink and take drugs. After many months of work and a number of crises, the woman agreed to try moving into a care home. In many respects the move was a success – her health improved greatly, she seemed generally to like living there and she appreciated the fact that she felt safer than at home. In spite of this, the outcome of the intervention was not transformative. As the social worker herself said:

> I suppose the only way I would have felt completely happy with it is if at the last review she'd have said 'this place is really great – I'm really, really happy'. But she didn't say that, she said 'when's my next glass of sherry?'

There may also be situations in which a social worker is seen as helpful by one person (perhaps a exhausted carer), but interfering by someone else (the person they care for who is persuaded to accept help from outside the family). Often, when working with adults who have the mental capacity to make their own decisions, social workers' influence is limited. We may try to do everything we can to establish a relationship with someone and work with them to improve their situation, but 'relationship' is a two-way business and sometimes it is not possible to reach a satisfactory outcome. Some situations remain intractable and different people's views about what should happen can be irreconcilable. In such circumstances even the best social worker may be unable to find common ground or a 'negotiated accommodation of perceptions' (Hugman, 2003, p. 1031). If in the case we have just mentioned, the woman had decided not to stay in residential care, but had gone home and continued to be abused by her family, would that have made the social work any less good? The eventual outcome of our work is often not directly within our control, but depends on both the people we are working with and the quality of the care services provided.

Outcomes are clearly important and if social workers never made a positive difference, there would be no point to the profession at all. However, it is very difficult to measure outcomes in a meaningful way – to capture the detail of an improved relationship and a sense of having been listened to and understood, or to estimate the extent to which a move into residential care has been welcomed or accepted. The reports produced by standardised, computerised data will always be very much cruder than this. So, while not denying the importance of the outcome, the best practice approach also emphasises the somewhat unfashionable value of concentrating on process. Whatever the outcome, the way in which social work is done can have a transformative effect, so that people feel understood, supported to make decisions and helped to think through difficulties and make plans.

Telling stories: exposing and learning from practice

By listening in detail to the ways in which social workers talk about and make sense of their practice, and using these accounts as the basis of our writing, we are essentially taking a narrative approach. Social workers themselves spend a lot of time trying to make sense of situations by giving them a shape or a 'narrative' – often bringing together many different and contradictory perspectives. Writing assessments, having supervision or holding safeguarding meetings are all about trying to make sense of complex realities. However, this narrative-making is generally hidden (unless something goes horribly wrong), taking place in the homes of clients and the heads of social workers as they try to make sense of what they have heard. As Adams et al. (2009, p. 8) have said, this reflection, or thoughtfulness, 'should be the six-sevenths of the iceberg of practice lying below the surface', and social workers need to be constantly aware that the way in which they think can have a profound effect on the decisions that are eventually made. The best practice approach adopted in this book makes some of the thinking process itself visible, so that we can both critique and learn from it. As Rita Wilder Craig (2007, p. 434) quotes in an article on personal narrative and hospital social work:

> Life needs more exposing. If anyone has a chance to contribute to the exposé, I say take it. (Weingarten, 1997, p. xii)

In our view, making practice visible in this way is one of the most powerful and thought-provoking ways of learning. A story does not tell you what you need to know or do; it is not prescriptive, but it does invite you to respond. In Frank's words, stories are not

> models of correct responses to dilemmas, told so that others can act in similar ways in similar situations ... If they are models of anything, the stories model moral sensitivity to what makes each situation unique and each decision difficult. (Frank, 2004, p. 7)

The reader is drawn in to engage with the dilemmas and difficulties faced and is encouraged to ask 'What do I think? What would I have done?'

Much of the richness of the stories in this book comes from the ways in which practitioners describe their practice. Those of us who teach students in universities spend a lot of time telling them to analyse rather than simply describe. However, in the best practice approach, we are promoting the value of real description, from real practitioners, in order to make good day-to-day practice visible and capture the 'adventures and atmospheres' that are so often lacking in accounts of social work (Ferguson, 2010, p. 1102). For us, that means writing well, avoiding jargon and drawing out the human experiences and dilemmas at the heart of social work in ways that are imaginatively engaging for the reader.

Finding our voice

It has always been difficult for social workers to describe exactly what they do in objective terms, because so much depends on the people and situations they encounter. In the following 12 case studies alone, social workers can be found negotiating with a landlord, arguing for funding, trying to educate a care agency, taking part in professionals' meetings, calming people's anger and anxiety, exercising legal powers under the Mental Capacity Act 2005 and buying a laundry basket. The variety and practicality of many of the tasks militates against easy definition and in formal, organisational terms, all of these activities would be swept up under the umbrella of 'care management', often with little recognition of the actual work involved. However, the truth is that the extraordinary variety, the humanity and the understanding that the most ordinary thing (a laundry basket) can make an enormous difference is one of social work's greatest strengths.

Jennifer Osmond and Ian O'Connor (2004) write helpfully about the 'formalising of the unformalised' in an article based on their research into the way social workers communicate knowledge in practice. Like other researchers before them, they found that practitioners rarely use the same language as academics to talk about their practice. Explicit theories are often echoed, the knowledge communicated is frequently speculative, informal and unlabelled; metaphor is common. Similarly, the social workers we listened to in writing this book did not generally use the language of assessment, risk management, personalisation or empowerment. They rarely, if ever, mentioned Codes of Practice or even legislation, although it was clear that this was known and largely internalised. Agency policy and procedure was also known and worked with – sometimes as something to be manipulated or creatively circumvented. Instead, they talked about complex relationships, challenging dilemmas and difficult decisions. We were reminded of Ann Weick's assertion that

> [t]he profession's first voice is found most fully in what we have come to call practice wisdom, the accumulation of knowledge that is flavoured with the richness and intricacies of years of collective practice experience. (Weick, 2000, p. 400)

Perhaps what is at the heart of the best practice approach we are advocating here is an attempt to give a platform to this 'first voice', with which social workers talk about what they do with clarity and confidence. It is not a voice that is often heard in public and bears little relation to the language used by politicians, managers and policy makers as they focus on tasks, targets, effectiveness and efficiency. With this 'official' language so dominant, it is unsurprising that social workers sometimes think about themselves and their work in these terms, creating all the more need for the 'first voice' to be heard and for it to critique and challenge the dominant discourse.

Despite the criticism, the managerialism and the 'deficit culture', what comes out most forcefully in the accounts in this book is the social workers' enjoyment of and belief in what they do. Our hope is that this confidence can inspire more coherent ways for social workers and educators to think, write and talk publicly about social work, based on a collective understanding of its real strengths and achievements.

Part 1

Relationships

2 Relationships

Introduction

In the chapters that follow, we explore the highly skilled practice of three experienced social workers as they each demonstrate the central importance of the social worker's relationship with the client through their humane, compassionate and respectful practice. The work described here gives us a great deal to be optimistic about and much to learn from. The social workers we spoke to were full of energy and enthusiasm for their profession, while the commitment they displayed towards their clients was striking. This is not to suggest that social work which places relationships at its core is either easy to achieve or unconstrained by the context of current practice. In fact each of the social workers we talked to spoke of their unease about the current and future state of social work. We heard, for example, about the necessity of 'tweaking the system' and 'going under the radar' in order to achieve the quality of practice that was aspired to. A recurring theme was the increasing difficulty of 'getting away with' spending as much time as was needed on any single case. All three expressed concern about what they saw as moves towards increasingly brief and prescriptive approaches to practice. These trends were unanimously seen as a threat to the kind of relationship-based practice that the social workers had found to be both effective and highly valued by older people and carers. Some of the issues that this situation raises will be discussed in more detail in the next section. In this chapter and in the three that follow however, the focus is on the skilled approaches to relationship building that were at the heart of a series of successful practice interventions.

Taking Time

When working with people and their needs, emotional work is rarely quick work. (Howe, 2008, p. 190)

As David Howe suggests, relationships take time to establish and social work that explicitly draws on the relationship between the social worker and the client cannot be rushed. As a way of working, this clearly has resource implications. Helen Gorman (2000) argues rightly that the tension between welfare objectives and resource constraints is probably felt more acutely in adult social care than in any other area. The social workers we spoke to were mindful of this demand and maintained a realistic awareness of the limited resources available within their agencies to meet the needs of large numbers of people. However they were also able to make critical and considered judgements about how their own time as part of a scarce resource should be spent.

In all three cases, the social workers argued for the importance of working at the pace of their clients rather than in response to an externally imposed deadline. Additional time was felt to be needed in order to build relationships that would enable helpful work to take place. Without the insights made possible by these relationships, the quality of life experienced by the older people involved would almost certainly have been significantly and even dangerously diminished. The investment of time was therefore seen as an important preventative measure. Len and Nina, who you will read about in Chapter 5, would have faced significantly greater risk without numerous small interventions over a long period of time on the part of their social worker. Similarly, if John, the carer in Chapter 4 had felt less able to be honest with his social worker, the pressure on him and the consequent danger to his wife could only have continued to intensify.

Perhaps the most important means by which the relationships in these stories developed was through talk. Patient, careful and skilled interactions led by social workers helped to overcome initial feelings of hostility or mistrust on the part of the people they were working with. In all three cases, these early relational difficulties were worked through and replaced by constructive, trusting relationships. However, as Nigel Parton points out, talking offers more than a means of establishing strong relationships, it is also 'the way we understand and come to terms with difficult and painful experiences' (Parton, 2003, p. 3). In each of these situations, talk was central to the social work intervention and was used by clients and carers to share difficult and painful aspects of their lives, echoing Parton's further observation:

> Users say clearly that what they value is the experience of talking which helps them to make sense of their experience and which gives them the

opportunity to better control and cope with their life and try to change it accordingly. (Parton, 2003, p. 3)

Furthermore, talking characterised by close, empathic listening on the part of the social workers was the basis on which professional judgements were made, decisions taken and ways forward agreed with clients and carers. The time taken to talk is therefore significant as both a therapeutic method and a tool for practical action and decision making.

Depth, not surface engagement

A number of social work commentators have suggested that the current bureaucratic climate in social work is antagonistic towards in-depth interventions, favouring instead a superficial kind of practice which marginalises thinking and feeling and privileges doing (Wilson et al., 2011). While it is difficult to deny the general truth of this assertion, it is also clear that the practice described in the following chapters was anything but superficial or bureaucratic. It was characterised rather by a strong inclination towards in-depth relationships as the medium through which practitioners engage with the complexity and uniqueness of human experience. David Howe expresses this eloquently:

When reason demands logic and detachment, the human spirit thrives on involvement, relationships and a determination to embrace the tangle of experience. (Howe, 2008, p. 194)

It was evident from the enthusiasm and care with which the social workers we talked to spoke about their practice that they were deeply engaged with the complexity and detail of their clients' unique situations. This engagement with individual biography (Tanner and Harris, 2008) and the 'interpretive angles' that people take on their own experiences (Saleeby, 2006, p. 16) is at the heart of relationship-based practice. It might appear self-evident that good social work involves caring about people's lives and being interested in what happens to them. However, this depth of involvement can too easily be lost in the undeniably bureaucratic and technological frameworks of community care practice. As Rachel, whose practice is described in the next chapter put it:

Sometimes you're so busy that it's tempting to just go through the motions – ask the questions on the form, feed the computer, arrange the service and *hope the outcome is ok. But the practice you'd describe as 'best', the practice you're proud of because it makes a real difference to service users, happens when you take the time to really find out what's going on for people.*

Rachel often had to be quite determined in her work with Michael in order to move beyond his initial account of particular events or experiences and establish a more real and honest understanding of his situation. There is a fine line in social work between being intrusive and recognising when it is in the interests of the services user to persist in seeking a more frank and open interaction. Some of the older people and their carers with whom social workers have contact will be very clear about their needs and the sort of help they are looking for. In such cases the process of assessment and the establishment of entitlement will probably be very straightforward. Showing respect in these circumstances may precisely mean *not* intruding too deeply into people's personal situations. At other times however, best practice may involve social workers in exercising a sort of 'compassionate scepticism' about what they are first being told and questioning initial or surface versions of events offered by those with whom they are working. The extent to which such exploration beneath the surface is possible or desirable is of course dependent on the situation and is a matter of skilled professional judgement.

Where there are issues of abuse or other safeguarding concerns, the process of discovering as much as possible about a situation from the perspective of everyone concerned is a necessity, legitimated by clear policy guidance. There are however many other circumstances and many understandable reasons why people who use (or refuse) social services are less than open about their lives and needs. All the older people described in this section were proud, resourceful and independent and all had good reason not to fully trust state authorities. In spite of this, in all three cases their vulnerability, isolation and level of need was lessened by a caring social worker who persisted in the building of a relationship leading to more openness and better understanding of the needs of the individuals involved. The social workers moved slowly, building up trust and, with it, people's willingness to reveal more about their lives. In each case, the work that took place involved the exercise of respectful, compassionate professional judgement and appropriate use of authority.

The depth of engagement shown by social workers in the following chapters was characterised not only by their observable relational skills, but by their strong imaginative, empathetic involvement with the experiences they were encountering. Hanley (2009, p. 178) defines empathy as 'a sense of sharing emotions, feelings and experiences with another person'. Kroll (2010, p. 78), drawing on Shulman (1999) and Trevithick (2005), suggests the more precise 'capacity to feel *with* someone, show some understanding of these feelings and put them into words'. She contrasts this with 'sympathy, where you feel *for* someone, moved by another's pain'.

An approach to social work which places empathy and relationship building at its heart is perceptibly different in emphasis from practice which focuses predominantly on issues of empowerment and choice. While the latter resonates strongly with current policy and practice, it may be that choice is not the most pressing concern for many of the most frail and vulnerable older users of social services. Pamela Trevithick (2003) suggests that practical and emotional responses are in fact difficult to separate in work with people experiencing extreme frailty. Consistency and reliability for those whose lived experience is dominated by dependency inevitably becomes an emotional, not just a practical concern. All three social workers in this section of the book sought and achieved practical solutions which increased people's choices and gave them greater control over their lives. However, they all also engaged deeply with the experiences and emotions of those they were working with, including their feelings of frailty, dependency and vulnerability. As Amanda Grenier (2006, p. 299) points out:

> Understanding and addressing the emotional aspects of what professionals know as 'frailty' may improve the likelihood of appropriate professional responses to older persons.

In all three situations, it is difficult to imagine how the positive practical outcomes, which were greatly valued by the clients themselves, would have been possible without a high degree of empathy and imaginative engagement on the part of the social workers involved.

Professional judgement and use of authority

In their research into effective social work relationships, de Boer and Coady (2007, p. 35) found that clients value both 'a humanistic attitude and style' and a 'soft, mindful and judicious use of power'. In the three chapters which follow and indeed in the stories of social work done well throughout this book, careful use of power, authority and professional judgement emerge as core components of skilled practice. Again and again, we see that social workers who are deeply concerned with improving the situations of older people are figures of strength and sources of advice as well as promoters of independence and choice. The building of a relationship of confidence and trust between the client and the social worker is the foundation which enables support and guidance to be offered and received in a spirit of authenticity and genuine helpfulness.

Each of the older people and carers in this section was able to exercise considerable choice and control over their own lives or had someone close to them to make choices on their behalf. In spite of this evident capacity to make independent decisions, it would be difficult to argue that the guidance and advice of the social worker did not significantly improve the safety, comfort and well-being of those concerned. In other situations, particularly those involving very frail and vulnerable older people, the exercise of professional judgement to guide and help with decision making may be even more necessary and central to the practice which takes place.

Adult social care policy in the UK has for some time been moving towards a more 'personalised' approach which promotes the independence and choice of the client (Great Britain, Department of Health, 2005, 2007a). For the current government this means individuals being treated as capable, competent citizens, able to choose and control their own care (Great Britain, Department of Health, 2010c, DH, 2012a). The aspiration to develop a more flexible, responsive service that values people's expertise is both welcome and overdue. However, some commentators have cautioned that current social care policies risk the development of a culture within which choice and control are promoted uncritically in all situations. As Liz Lloyd (2006, p. 1180) points out, social workers are often involved when older people are at their most vulnerable and dependant and when their capacity for choice and autonomy have been shattered:

> At such times it is difficult to see how the rational exercise of choice and control is viable or desirable...

Lloyd is not suggesting here that frail, older people do not have the right to make choices about their lives, but rather that a caring and empathetic response may not involve prioritising or promoting choice above other concerns. She continues:

Assumptions about older people's readiness to assume a position in a process of rational decision making can be counterproductive. In such circumstances, care is required, which acknowledges the effect of shattering events and allows the older person time to recover.

In such situations skills in building humane, compassionate relationships, which respect people's vulnerability and need for care, may be valued more by the older person concerned than the promotion of choice and autonomy. The expertise, guidance and professional judgement of the social worker in these circumstances is vital.

Use of self

When asked to evaluate the help they have received, clients and carers tend to talk about their social workers largely in terms of their personal qualities. Warmth and friendliness come up time and again as highly rated attributes in research studies into client experience (Howe, 1993, p. 2008). It should hardly be a surprise that people value many of the same qualities in their social workers as they do in their other relationships. It is however an important truth to reaffirm at a time when many would agree with Mark Lymbery's assertion that social work with older people has become

> a highly routinised, bureaucratised process where the emphasis has been to 'resolve' needs as quickly and as cost effectively as possible. (Lymbery, 2005, p. 181)

The three social workers whose practice you will read about shortly shared many skills and similarities of approach, including a belief in the importance of their relationship with their client. They were however a long way from the sort of 'detached' and 'interchangeable' professional (Parton, 2003, p. 11) suggested by Lymbery's analysis above. Sarah, Rachel and Eric – the social workers in the following chapters – were strongly aware of the increasingly bureaucratic context in which they were working. In spite of the tendency towards uniformity and routine which characterises this trend however, they were each able to bring a striking degree of distinctiveness and personal commitment to the relationships they told us about.

The way individual personalities and personal choices informed the practice we are showcasing here raises the question of how far good social work is intuitive or dispositional. While much of the knowledge

21

that informs practice can clearly be taught or learnt through experience, some of what makes social workers stand out as 'best' may be innate. Stephen Webb is one of those who suggests that people who choose to become social workers generally want to do the best that they can for others. This may sound obvious, but Webb's key point is that codes and prescriptions for practice are insufficient when it comes to the promotion of ethical social work. He argues rather that 'practising values and believing in them are acts of an ethical disposition or will' (Webb, 2006, p. 202) or, put another way, that the 'ethical identity of social work is dispositional rather than functional' (Webb, 2006, p. 214).

The central assertion of this chapter is that the relationship between the social worker and their client is at the heart of good practice. If this is accepted, then it seems likely that the personal strengths, flaws and inclinations of all those involved, including the social worker, will impact on the processes and outcomes of practice. This is not to suggest that good social work has no need for a wide range of practical and theoretical knowledge. It is rather to propose that the very best practice also draws on the innate personal characteristics of the individual worker. Yelloly and Henkel (1995, p. 7) liken this to the skill of a musician:

> It is likely that the effective worker, like the accomplished musician, combines an informed understanding of principles and theories with an intuitive gift which enables her to tune in to the experiences of troubled people.

In most cases the knowledge base of the social workers we talked to was clearly evident, but all they tended to downplay the skills involved in their interventions. This may have been due not only to modesty, but to the fact that these skills were partly intuitive and dispositional. A lot of the social workers' choices were made because they cared about the people they were working with. This often involved interventions which need to be understood not only in terms of professional codes of practice and values, but also as an individual, personal response to people and situations.

The ability to combine personal intuition and informed understanding in an effective use of self means that social workers need to be aware of their own feelings and responses and able to reflect on them. Some writers have framed this capacity in terms of 'emotional intelligence':

> Social and health care work is emotional work of a high order whether it's with older people, children and families, offenders, disabled children and adults or the mentally ill. The more intelligent practitioners are about emotions and the part they play in health and health care work, the more

sensitive, thoughtful and effective will be their practice. Emotional intelligence is therefore a core skill without which practice would not only be ineffective, it would lack humanity. (Howe, 2008, pp. 1–2)

As Howe suggests, the ability to be intelligent about their own emotions means that practitioners are more likely to be available and responsive to the emotions of older people and carers. This 'capacity to handle both one's own and others' emotions effectively' (Morrison, 2007, p. 245) necessitates a high degree of self-awareness. We have suggested that the responses of the social workers in the following chapters to the people and the circumstances they encountered incorporated a personal and therefore an emotional dimension. If this had not been accompanied by a well-developed self-awareness, however, the social workers would have risked getting 'caught up' in what Wilson et al. (2011, p. 21) call 'unhelpful "rescuing" or over-dependent relationships'. Responding emotionally to clients is not the same as responding with emotional intelligence. It is therefore essential that social workers are able to recognise and understand their own feelings in order to be able to use them effectively and appropriately for the benefit of those they are working with. This may be particularly relevant to work with older people. Most social workers will not routinely find themselves in situations similar to those they encounter in their professional lives. However, fears of their own frailty, vulnerability, aging and eventual death may provoke strong feelings in response to older people. Without a high degree of insight social workers may be blown around by their emotional reactions and unable to make the caring, yet fully informed professional judgements that are essential to good social work practice.

The self-awareness that involves social workers in 'acknowledging personal involvement' (Brechin, 2000, p. 29) in this way is associated with the concept of 'reflexive practice'. Adams et al. (2002, p. 3) define reflexivity as 'a circular process in which social workers "put themselves in the picture"' by recognising that they are changed by their experiences in practice and that as part of the same process, they influence and change others. All three social workers in this section spoke about what they had learnt from the particular practice interventions they described. More than this however, they were able to reflect on how they had been personally changed by their involvement in the lives of these particular clients. This is exemplified by Sarah, who reflects on her work with John and his wife Mary:

I'd worked with lots of people with dementia before and with lots of carers and I don't think I'd done a bad job, but I was more myself in this situation. It was definitely a two way process – they got a lot from having me involved and I got a lot from them. We sort of shifted things along together.

Conclusion

The social work practice described in the next three chapters features a series of humane, compassionate and respectful interventions on the part of the social workers involved. There are many aspects of the work that we could have drawn out for further discussion and learning, but the focus in this section of the book is on the relationship between the social worker and the client as a foundation for good practice. As we have seen, a number of key areas emerge as characteristic of skilled relationship-based practice.

Time is an important factor in enabling really constructive helping relationships to become established. In complex situations social workers need to move at people's own pace if they are to be trusted by those they are working with. This raises complex resource issues in a period when not only are finances constrained, but the number of older people in need of a social work service is rising. In such difficult times, it is particularly important that social workers are enabled to make clear professional judgements about how their particular skills and expertise should be used. Prevention is a stated priority for the current government (Great Britain, Department of Health, 2010c). Time taken to really understand the needs of older people at key points in their lives can lead to small-scale, early interventions which prevent the need for more expensive and potentially disempowering services at a later stage.

Another key theme is depth of engagement. Sometimes brief, straightforward interventions are appropriate in social work with older people. Not everyone will want or need to share their life story with a social worker. In less clear-cut situations however, responding imaginatively to the uniqueness and complexity of an older person's story will be essential to the genuine meeting of their needs. Sometimes an in-depth response will involve fine judgements about whether it is necessary to explore beneath the surface or seek to challenge a client's initial account of his or her needs. We have used the term compassionate scepticism to describe this highly skilled dimension of social work with older people.

Professional judgement and the helpful, caring and constructive use of authority also surface as recurring elements of good practice. Extreme vulnerability and frailty are often present in the lives of older people and while these experiences never define the whole person, they do need to be acknowledged and respected. Sometimes older people may be too unwell or too tired to engage fully with detailed choices and decisions about their care. In such situations the social work role may include wise and empathetic guidance and support in order to ensure the best possible outcome for the older person.

The final area identified as key to effective relationship-based practice is use of self. In the following chapters, three social workers – Rachel, Sarah and Eric – demonstrate the professional confidence to be able to draw on their own emotional responses and personalities as part of a helpful social work intervention. A reflexive, authentic and emotionally intelligent approach to social work with older people is vital to the development of honest and open relationships. Importantly, such an approach is also essential in enabling social workers themselves to remain in touch with their feelings and reactions to the often emotionally demanding situations they encounter.

3 Rachel and Michael: Careful Relationship Building

Questions to ask yourself as you read:

- Why do you think Rachel succeeded in building a successful relationship with Michael where others failed?
- What is an assessment?
- What made residential care such a positive outcome in this situation?

Rachel and Michael

When Michael was first referred to the older adults community team and allocated to Rachel, he was in his early seventies. According to the community psychiatric nurse (CPN) who made the referral, he had never had a mental health diagnosis, in spite of behaviour which some people regarded as 'odd', but presented rather as someone with a mild learning difficulty. Michael was retired at this point and had not worked for many years, although he would often talk about time spent in the army as a young man and about a series of casual jobs on farms and local holiday camps. He also spoke often about his hope that he would one day get married, in spite of seemingly never having had a long-term relationship.

The CPN had been involved for just over a year and made the referral because of Michael's increasing personal care needs. He had become incontinent of urine and faeces and in spite of medical investigations and treatment, this now seemed to be a permanent feature of his life.

Rachel made several joint visits to Michael with the CPN. Her hope was that accompanying a worker who had known Michael for some time would enable her to establish a relationship with him more quickly than would otherwise have been possible. In most situations,

Rachel would probably have been right, but Michael was someone whose instinctive wariness and difficult life experiences made it hard for him to trust new people. In fact, as Rachel explains, the presence of two workers in his home only seemed to be making things worse:

I was getting nowhere. Michael didn't want to talk to me. He didn't see why he should trust me and I don't blame him – he was outnumbered by 'professionals' with their own agendas after all. All I was getting from him was a sense of frustration and disappointment.

Rachel decided that if she was going to make any progress with Michael she needed to take a step back and start the process of building a relationship again from the beginning:

I decided to visit Michael alone. I had some reservations because he was quite loud and a bit intimidating. He sometimes seemed like he might become aggressive, although there was nothing in his history to suggest that he presented a physical risk. I talked it over with my manager and we agreed that I should trust my instincts.

Rachel was right. Michael was much more inclined to open up to her during a one-on-one conversation than he had been when she was accompanied by another professional:

It wasn't that the CPN was doing anything wrong, it was more that something more informal was needed. I had to stop thinking in terms of doing an assessment and think more about getting to know Michael. I felt I could do that better without a third person there. Maybe that says as much about me as about him. Anyway, it worked.

Michael was someone who could easily have slipped between services. Although he had some mental health needs and a degree of learning disability, he did not easily meet the eligibility criteria or thresholds of entitlement to a service. A less careful adult care social worker than Rachel or one more prepared to take situations at face value might easily have missed the extent of his needs.

In fact as Rachel got to know Michael, she found that he was almost completely socially isolated. His parents were long dead and he had no contact with any other family members. He had no friends, and neighbours tended to avoid him because of the strong smell of urine in his flat and about his person. People he met were wary of Michael's loud and rather chaotic manner of speaking, which could easily be interpreted as aggression.

Rachel, who is a naturally quiet and describes herself as an instinctively tidy person, did not find any of this easy either. She described Michael's flat as

> incredibly cluttered – the worst I've seen actually... He found it hard to throw anything away – ever, so it had become very difficult to move around and impossible to keep clean. I broached the possibility of making changes once or twice and found that this was clearly a touchy subject. In the end I felt the clutter and the mess were not really a priority. I wasn't in the business of trying to make Michael become someone he wasn't or trying to impose my own standards of hygiene.

After a while and following careful negotiation, Rachel was able to introduce the idea of help with personal care for Michael:

> As I got to know him, I realised that Michael would get frustrated when he felt other people were making decisions for him. Every time I introduced something new, I had to give him information and then space and time to reach his own conclusion. I told him about the help available with personal care without pushing it then I came back and asked him what sorts of things might make life better for him. Eventually we came to a shared agreement about what the right package of care would be.

Michael began to receive help from care workers each morning. While this did not transform his life, it did mean that his personal hygiene improved and that he was not shunned to the same extent by other people when he attended local coffee mornings or other social events.

The package of care Michael was receiving worked well for nearly two years. Although this would normally have been reviewed periodically by another team, Rachel successfully made a case to her manager do this herself because she understood how difficult Michael would find it to accept a new worker. This meant that Rachel was able to go on getting to know Michael and to continue to offer him some support. She talks about her growing ability to read Michael's mood and interpret his tone of voice and body language:

> He would get angry and frustrated about things. Sometimes it would be a bill or a letter, perhaps something in the flat that didn't work or the way someone had treated him. His anger was very internal – his speech would

get louder and his gestures more dramatic. I got to know him well enough to be able to ask what was wrong and he got to know me well enough to be able to tell me.

One day however, Rachel took a telephone call from the distressed owner of a seaside Bed and Breakfast (B and B), a short train ride from Michael's home. Michael had decided that he needed a holiday and had booked himself in to the B and B. The train ride was one that Michael had made many times in his life and was the only journey that he felt confident to make alone. Michael had stayed for one night and had been 'very incontinent' both in his own room and in the communal lounge. The proprietor of the B and B politely asked if Rachel could 'arrange for him to go home'. Rachel takes up the story:

> *Michael is a very big man and a very loud man. The B and B owner was clearly afraid to ask him to leave so I spoke to Michael on the phone. I didn't want to be dishonest, but I didn't want to upset or embarrass him either. I talked about the difficulty of climbing up and down the stairs at the B and B and about Michael not being able to have the support he was used to at home. Eventually, I suggested that he come back and we should look together at places for a break, which were nearer to home. I sent a taxi to collect Michael and arranged to visit him later that day.*

Rachel met with Michael as planned and as was usual during their conversations enabled him to come up with his own ideas about the kind of support he would need if he was to go away from home for a few days. As a result, Rachel managed to arrange a week's 'holiday' for Michael in a seaside residential home. She admits that the local authority funding panel took some persuading before they would agree to pay a contribution towards what was formally termed 'respite' care, but this was eventually agreed.

Michael enjoyed his week of respite. His willingness to use the walk in shower every day made a big difference to his personal hygiene and was probably one of the reasons why he seemed to have more success than usual interacting with staff members and with other residents.

> *That break did him a lot of good. He knew it had gone well and after the bed and breakfast fiasco, which could have been so demoralising, I think he ended up feeling a real sense of achievement about being able to socialise better than he'd managed for a long time.*

Michael's physical health was gradually declining however. He was now considerably less mobile than he had been when Rachel first got to know him and his eyesight was beginning to deteriorate. The care workers, who were still visiting Michael daily, began to report increasing episodes of evident distress and frustration on his part. Rachel was in the process of reassessing Michael's needs with a view to an increased package of care, when he was diagnosed with cataracts and being in urgent need of an operation on both eyes.

Rachel was concerned about Michael returning to his flat after his operation, but she knew from now long experience that any alternative solution would need to come from Michael himself:

> *I got him to think about what it would be like when he got home and what sorts of difficulties he might have, then very gradually we moved on to what we might do to help. Eventually he came up with the suggestion of going back to the place where he had been for respite.*

Michael spent two weeks in the residential home after the operation on one eye. When he got back to his flat he told Rachel that for the first time in his life he had felt that no one saw him as different from everyone else. Rachel was therefore not surprised that Michael was enthusiastic about returning to the home after the operation on his other eye, nor that he then asked if he could stay permanently.

Michael's care needs were now such that he easily met the criteria for residential care and fortunately the home had a bed available.

Rachel knew that if the transition to permanent residential care was to work, she would have to work closely with staff in the home to help them get to know Michael and understand his moods and responses. She achieved this initially by writing a detailed care plan and by taking time to discuss his needs in detail with senior care staff and to facilitate conversations with Michael and his key worker. Michael has now been living at the home for nearly a year and Rachel talks with evident enthusiasm about the success of the move:

> *He really enjoys the routine and he says he feels at home because no one bullies him. For the first time in all the years I've known him, Michael seems to have a sense of identity. He's become very much part of the home – he's a strong advocate for the other residents. His incontinence is still a problem, but he manages it with help, far better than he ever did at home. Of course there are still difficult times. The staff are learning that Michael's grumpiness is not a sign of aggression, but a way of saying that something is wrong. Sometimes*

they call me and I visit because he probably will still talk to me more openly than to anyone else. His relationship with the care staff is improving all the time though – I don't think he'll need me much in the future.

Discussion

Rachel says that she chose to talk about her work with Michael mainly because she felt that the conclusion was so successful. For many older people, the move to a residential or nursing home is unwelcome and represents an unwanted loss of independence. For Michael however, residential care seems to have provided some of the stability, security and social opportunities that were missing when he lived alone. While Rachel acknowledges that there is an element of chance in this successful result, it is also clear that the relationship she built with Michael was central to the process and to the outcome of her practice in this case.

Starting with her initial decision to visit Michael alone, Rachel recognised that finding a way to establish a mutually respectful, understanding relationship, was an essential prerequisite if they were to work together effectively. Again and again, research has shown that the relationship between social workers and their clients is the key to successful interventions (Howe, 1993; Wilson et al., 2011). The recurring themes which clients identify as most important in their dealings with social workers are summarised succinctly by David Howe as "accept me, understand me, and talk with me" (Howe, 1993, p.139). Rachel was able to acknowledge and also to see beyond Michael's initial hostility and frustration and try a different approach to building an effective relationship with him.

Rachel's work with Michael did not always conform to procedures that might have been expected by her employing agency. For example, carrying out a joint assessment with the CPN could have been effective and helpful in another situation, but in this case, Rachel recognised that it would be better for her to visit Michael alone. She argued successfully to keep the case open, rather than passing it to someone else to review as was usual in Rachel's team, while arranging respite care as a hurried response to Michael's own disastrous holiday arrangements, rather than as the planned result of an assessment was a creative and humane response, rather than a procedural one.

Many commentators have argued against the trend in social work towards highly proceduralised ways of working with an emphasis on measurable competencies (Jordan, 2001; Morrison, 2007; Wilson

31

et al., 2011) and the calculation of risk (Kemshall, 2002; Webb, 2006). Certainly, the work which is felt to be good by social workers in this book tends to place relationships with their clients at the heart of practice and often finds creative ways of working with or even around agency procedures. As David Howe maintains:

> Social work and social care are essentially relationship-based practices even if many of the explicit techniques and statutory demands impose more formal rules of engagement. (Howe, 2008, p. 181)

None of Rachel's actions were undertaken without the consent of her managers, but her skill in this case, was to recognise when she needed to push at the boundaries of the social work role as defined by her employer. Michael was an unusual man with a complex personality and sometimes unpredictable interpersonal responses. The relationship that Rachel established and the reciprocal understanding this created gave her confidence about the most effective ways of meeting Michael's needs. Rachel's practice was therefore considered, compassionate and deeply respectful of Michael's feelings in a way which would have been difficult to achieve through a more routine or procedural approach. As Rachel herself said,

> [i]t took a while for Michael and I to get used to each other. I was feeling my way and looking for ways to get to know him and understand him better. I had to take it at his pace and respond to his agendas, so the conventional idea of 'doing and assessment' was really in the background.

Rachel's creative and flexible response to agency procedure was mirrored in the reflective approach which underpinned her work with Michael. In common with many of the social workers who appear in this book, Rachel did not feel that she used an identifiable theoretical or methodological approach. Her practice in this case was informed by psychosocial insights into Michael's seemingly aggressive manner, his social isolation and his need to feel a sense of belonging. It was also unquestionably person-centred and anti-oppressive in its attempt to empower Michael and to facilitate genuine choice. Above all however, Rachel demonstrated a consistent and conscious ability to reflect on her practice.

Jan Fook argues that the ability to take a holistic perspective is a defining characteristic of the reflective practitioner who 'must take into account all factors which impinge on the situation at any given time' (2002, p. 40). In other words, reflection allows practitioners to use the totality of their knowledge in relation to specific events and situations in order to develop their own theories for practice. As a reflective practitioner, Rachel was able to use the insights she gained as she got to know Michael and his unique circumstances, to establish a specific and situated approach to practice in this case.

Nigel Parton draws on Donald Schön's (1987, 1991) theory of reflection to explain how practitioners 'construct and re-frame' their knowledge about situations through their relationships with their clients:

> Real world problems do not come well formed but, on the contrary, present themselves as messy and indeterminate. 'Knowing' in such situations is invariably *tacit* and *implicit*. It develops from dialogues with people about the situation through which the practitioner can come to understand the uniqueness, uncertainty and potential value conflicts that must be addressed and thereby reaches 'a new theory of the unique case' that informs action. (Parton, 2003, p. 2)

Rachel was able to draw on her own intuition and years of accumulated professional wisdom and knowledge in order to build the theory which informed her actions:

> *I was trying to get to a point where I could read Michael's manner and behaviour better and pick up the cues about when it was ok to probe more and when a topic was really out of bounds. There were also times when some quite firm recommendations were needed from me. I had to learn how to make that feel ok for Michael and recognise my own reaction, which was instinctively to feel a bit intimidated by him.*

One of the things that Rachel demonstrates here is an ability to interpret Michael's emotions while remaining aware of the feelings and responses that this provokes in her. She was therefore able to situate herself within the context of the particular episode of practice and to factor this understanding into her approach (Fook, 2002). Rachel's capacity to work constructively with her own and with Michael's feelings embodied the sort of emotional intelligence that is essential to relationship-based practice. David Howe defines this ability as 'a core skill, without which practice would not only be ineffective, it would lack humanity' (Howe, 2008, p. 2).

Michael's sometimes loud and angry way of communicating, which Rachel recognised as a sign of distress, was as far as it could be from her natural way of being. His isolation, chaotic lifestyle and often unhygienic home surroundings were miles away from the sorts of choices she would ever make in her own life. It was therefore essential for Rachel to

33

engage imaginatively and intelligently with Michael's emotional world in order to find points of genuine contact. This involved an awareness and questioning of her own instinctive responses which Rachel found challenging. Nevertheless she managed to communicate her genuine interest in Michael, in a way that was both respectful and supportive and led him to trust her. It is doubtful that a less emotionally intelligent practitioner would have responded so sensitively to the disastrous Bed and Breakfast incident or achieved such a positive outcome. However, Rachel was not only able to facilitate Michael's safe return home, she also made possible an alternative which benefitted his physical and emotional health and was sensitive to his deep need to make his own decisions and retain control over his own life.

Rachel describes the work she undertook with Michael, his key worker and other care staff to prepare for his permanent move to the residential home as 'the easiest part of my work with Michael'. Residential care was after all a positive choice for Michael and he was actively looking forward to it. However, the relationship that Rachel had built with Michael and the 'communication bridge' (Kadushin, 1990, p. 36) that had been established between them was undoubtedly an important factor in making this process 'easy'. Without Rachel's careful preparatory work and her insight into to the importance of her role as an advocate or 'bridge' between the residential home staff and Michael, his final move might have been far less straightforward.

In common with much work involving older people, this was a fluid and changing situation to which Rachel responded with emotional intelligence and good decision making, based on reflective practice, intuition, knowledge and experience. The relationship between Rachel and Michael was at the heart of the social work practice described here and it was this which made possible a series of sensitive and empathic interventions on Rachel's part. Her work with Michael was also characterised by an emphasis on process rather than simply on outcomes. In fact, the outcome for Michael was strikingly and, in some ways, unexpectedly positive, but this was achieved through a gradual process negotiated through the medium of a strengthening relationship of trust and a growing mutual understanding.

Nigel Parton argues that the most important skills social workers bring to their work are primarily those of 'knowing how' as opposed to 'knowing that' (Parton, 2003, p. 10). At the heart of Rachel's practice here was the skill of knowing how to build a humane, compassionate and respectful relationship, which enabled her to respond helpfully and appropriately to events in Michael's life as they occurred.

4 Sarah, John and Mary: A Carer under Pressure

Questions to ask yourself as you read:

- How does John and Mary's story challenge assumptions about the role of 'carer'?
- Why do you think John was so reluctant to accept help?
- Is it alright to like some clients more than others?

Sarah, John and Mary

The story below follows Sarah in her work with John and Mary. Like Rachel in the previous chapter, Sarah had to overcome initial hostility in order to build relationships that would enable her to make a difference to the lives of those she was working with. The relational dynamics and needs involved in this situation are very different from those discussed in Chapter 3. Here too however, the humane, compassionate and respectful relationships at the centre of Sarah's work offer an important contribution to an understanding of what is 'best' in practice with older people.

Having been appointed as an 'acting senior social worker' within the older adults team where she had worked for several years, Sarah was looking forward to taking on some more complex and challenging cases. She knew that John, a former college lecturer in his late seventies, had been caring for his wife Mary at home for a number of years. Mary had a diagnosis of severe rheumatoid arthritis and advanced dementia. She had been receiving services for some time, but now there were concerns from Mary's general practitioner (GP) and from the care agency involved in helping John to look after her that the situation was becoming increasingly precarious and risky.

Sarah telephoned John to make an appointment to visit and received an unexpectedly angry and hostile response:

He was furious to be telephoned out of the blue by 'yet another new worker'. He told me I was the third social worker to call him in the past six months and no one had 'bothered' to actually come and visit...

...He was right of course. We'd had a number of staff changes, for reasons which weren't in our control, but that didn't alter the fact that he'd had a lousy service. He was right to be angry and I should have recognised the situation from his point of view. Instead I phoned him without any warning, brightly offering a visit and expecting him to be pleased.

In spite of this difficult beginning, Sarah was able to agree with John that she would visit him and his wife at home a few days later:

As soon as I walked in, I could see that the level of care was very intense. Mary had her bed in the sitting room, there was a hoist, a commode and lots of other equipment around. Mary was able to make sounds, including occasional snatches of song, but she didn't really respond when I greeted her and she seemed to have very little independent movement.

Sarah's first visit to John and Mary lasted for more than two hours. John told her that a package of care had been arranged a year earlier, following Mary's most recent hospital admission. Day care had been organised three times a week in a local nursing home, but John had stopped this early on as it seemed to be making Mary distressed. A local care agency had been contracted to visit twice a day to help Mary get washed and ready for the day and to put her to bed at night. This was continuing, although John was unhappy with the timing and nature of the care being provided, and felt particularly aggrieved as the couple were paying for this themselves from their savings.

An assessment by an occupational therapist meant that Mary and John had been provided with a range of equipment, including the hoist which enabled Mary to be lifted in and out of bed, a commode and a special chair. There was a lot of other equipment in the house, much of it now discarded, which John had bought himself in an attempt to improve his wife's comfort and mobility.

He was very isolated and badly needed someone to talk to. Although there had been quite a bit of practical help provided, he felt he had been left without much real support or guidance. Problems were mounting up and he didn't know which way to turn next. He was also scared that if it looked as though he wasn't coping, Mary would have to go into a nursing home and he really didn't want that. At first he seemed very angry with everyone who'd been involved in Mary's care, but actually it was more frustration with the hitches and problems and the fact that the support they were getting wasn't more effective.

Following her first visit to Mary and John, Sarah spent a lot of time talking to other professionals and care staff who had been or who continued to be involved in supporting them. She found that the amount of care being provided by the private care agency had been changed and increased on a number of occasions in response to Mary's rapidly decreasing mobility. Some of the equipment provided when Mary had left hospital no longer met her needs and in some cases John had bought new equipment himself, which was also not quite right for Mary and had consequently lain unused in the house. The day care which had been set up partly to give John a break and to enable him to do household jobs such as shopping and meal preparation had been discontinued at an early stage. This left him struggling to manage day-to-day tasks and virtually unable to leave the house.

Sarah described the situation as

[a] patchwork of care that had been put together quite carefully, but which had rapidly come apart without anyone really noticing.

Staff changes in the community care team, where Sarah worked, meant that the package of care had not been reviewed as thoroughly as it should have been. The several temporary social workers to whom Mary's case was allocated, had seen in John, an active, capable and articulate man, who was in a position to fund his wife's care. He had sometimes expressed anger and dissatisfaction with the service he and his wife were receiving, but in his anxiety to ensure that Mary should not be moved to a nursing home, he had also assured those involved that he was managing the situation.

In fact, as Sarah developed a clearer picture of how John and Mary had been coping, it emerged that John had been taking increasing risks in order to maintain the situation at home. As Mary was no longer attending day care, he would rush out to the local supermarket to stock up on food while Mary was asleep, hoping that she would not wake and try to get up from the chair by herself. On one occasion he had returned to find Mary slumped over the side of the chair, unable to move. He had also developed a makeshift system of moving furniture against Mary's bed at night, so that she would not attempt to get out by herself and so risk falling.

In this situation, Sarah's intervention probably came just in time. John was only just managing to care for his wife, by taking risks which put her in danger of injuring herself and was becoming increasingly stressed and exhausted himself. Sarah began working with John to 'put the patchwork back together' by reassessing Mary's needs as well as his own needs as a carer.

It took ages to get the package right. We built up to three days a week day care in a local nursing home, but it had to be very gradual. He went with her at first and I had to do quite a bit of negotiation around him being allowed to help to care for her. She found it hard to settle for the first few months, especially when he wasn't there. I had to work quite hard to persuade him not to give up and stop the day care arrangement, but we all persevered and she's fine there now. It also makes a massive difference to him of course, because he can get things done at home and even have a bit of time for himself.

The introduction of day care which provided respite for John as well as personal care for Mary made a big difference to their lives. As the relationship of trust between the couple and staff in the nursing home grew, Sarah was also able to arrange week long respite for Mary every few months, to allow John to get away to visit friends with whom he had previously lost touch. Sarah was also involved in numerous small interventions which had a big impact on John and Mary's lives. For example, she visited John and Mary when the care workers were in the house helping Mary to get up and return to bed in order to help facilitate a conversation about how this could be done in a way that everyone felt comfortable with.

As Sarah worked with John and Mary to help strengthen their relationships with those involved in providing care and support, she got to know them better herself. Sarah speaks about the non-verbal as well as the verbal signs from both of them that a relationship of increasing trust and confidence was being established:

He's quite a formal, very dignified man. At first he used to shake my hand. Now he pats me on the back and I touch him on the shoulder. I used to find it hard to communicate with Mary at all, but now she holds my hand – very quietly; it feels like a kind of acceptance...

He told me a lot about their lives. Mary had been a community nurse and quite a pioneer in her field. He laughed about how she'd want her care to be 'just right', but he also felt it very deeply. He was devoted to her and hated the term 'carer'. He said he was her husband and they were in this together 'for better or worse'. They didn't have any children, so it was very much just the two of them. They listened to a lot of music and it had an amazingly calming effect on her. Sometimes he would sing to her – it was lovely to see.

In talking about her work with John and Mary, Sarah was very open about her affection for both of them and talked a lot about how much she has learnt from John about what a caring relationship can be like.

Sarah worked closely with several other health and social care professionals as she assessed Mary's needs and helped to arrange services for her and John. This included a referral to the local community psychiatric nursing team, which proved to be particularly beneficial for Mary. Although John had turned away this sort of specialist input in the past, Sarah was able to help him accept that this would now be a good thing for Mary.

The CPN was particularly good at communicating with Mary and helped to get her pain under control. Mary had arthritis and would rub parts of her body when they hurt. The CPN was able to suggest some techniques to John – things like the best sitting or lying positions for Mary and of course she was much calmer when she was experiencing less pain. I think it also helped John to see that he wasn't the only person who could help Mary or the only person who would want to.

As a senior social worker, Sarah often takes responsibility for the induction of new social workers into her organisation. On more than one occasion she has invited them to accompany her on visits to John and Mary:

It's a chance to show people how well the system can work when it all comes together. They are basically at the centre of the help they get and he has a lot of control over how services are delivered. Also John's happy to help by talking to new workers. It feels like we're on the same side now, whereas I think he used to feel that social services were the enemy.

Discussion

In common with many of the stories of social work done well that are included in this book, Sarah achieved a skilful balance between the relational and the practical dimensions of her work in this situation. The practical support that she was able to arrange made a substantial difference to the lives of both John and Mary. It is unlikely however that any change would have been as fully embraced or as effective in its outcome without the relationship of trust and confidence that Sarah was able to establish.

John and Mary had undoubtedly received a poor service in the months prior to Sarah's involvement. Social work appointments had been cancelled and promises of action had come to nothing. John's anger and disappointment had led him to become increasingly resistant to and mistrustful of outside intervention and more and more determined to find a way of coping with Mary's care by himself.

In order to make possible any future changes, Sarah needed to find ways of rebuilding John's trust in the support services available to him. She used herself and her own relational skills as a resource in this process:

> It's always tempting to go in and immediately start finding solutions, but I had to rewind quite a few steps with John and Mary. He needed to tell me about his anger – desperation really. That's not how he would have described it of course, but that's part of what I heard when he told me how it had been for the past few months. It was also really important to see them together. John was quite sharp and formal with me at first, but he was always incredibly gentle and caring with Mary.

Sarah's careful and sensitive approach involved listening, talking and learning about John and Mary's relationship as an effective foundation for her future work with them. The importance of talk as a way of enabling people to come to terms with and make sense of painful experiences is well documented (Parton and O'Byrne, 2000; Parton, 2003), but easily under-valued in social work with older people. This is an area of practice where the strong focus on assessing practical need and providing physical care can too easily lead workers to neglect the relationship between themselves and the people they are working with. Several recent commentators have argued that social work with adults and particularly with older people has become bureaucratic and managerial to a degree that eclipses the relational aspects of practice (Tanner and Harris, 2008; Postle, 2002). Others have referred to current trends in social work as 'de-humanising' (Howe, 2008, p. 193) and 'depersonalised' (Wilson et al., 2011, p. 7).

As we discussed in the previous chapter, evidence from research suggests that people who use services tend to evaluate social workers first and foremost in terms of their personal qualities (Howe, 1993; Webb, 2006) and that that the key ingredient of effective help is the professional relationship (Howe, 2008). This is not to suggest that practical outcomes are unimportant. No amount of talk can act as a substitute for a good night's sleep or the opportunity to take part in a valued hobby. In common with other social workers whose stories are told in this book however, Sarah recognised that the building of relationships in practice is a central component in the achievement of positive practical changes which can make a real difference to people's lives. As Veronica Coulshed (1991, p. 2) has pointed out:

> While it is true that people do not come to us looking for a relationship, and while it is no substitute for practical support, nevertheless we are one of the few groups who recognize the value of relating to others in a way which recognizes their experience as fundamental to understanding and action.

In John and Mary's case, several past assessments had taken place and services had been organised to meet a set of identified needs. It appears however that no one had really sought to understand the depth of John's anxiety about his wife's care or his ever-present fear that she might be removed to a nursing home against his will and hers. Nor had they recognised the extent to which his fears made him quick to find fault or to discontinue the help that had been put in place. By listening to John and responding to his concerns in a deeply humane and compassionate way, Sarah recognised that she needed to achieve John's trust in order to negotiate the kind of support that would really make a difference to him and to Mary. In this way, Sarah used her relational skills to achieve very real practical benefits that almost certainly enabled John and Mary to remain together for far longer than would otherwise have been possible.

John and Mary had quite substantial savings and had therefore been required to pay for most of the services, equipment and practical support they received. Sarah felt that this, along with John's articulate assurances that he could manage his wife's care on his own, helped to explain why they had received less attention from their local social services department than might be expected. Sarah explains:

> They were a bit overwhelmed by choice by the time I came along. John had been to a couple of shops selling mobility equipment because he knew he'd have to pay even if he went through the council. Some of what he bought just wasn't any use to Mary. He was also paying for more care than Mary needed at some times and not enough at others. The care workers actually gave him quite good advice about this, but at the time he was too anxious and cross to take it on board.

The need for people who pay for their own care to be given more help and advise with the often complex and expensive choices they have to make is supported by current government policy (Great Britain, Department of Health, 2010d). Nevertheless recent research suggests that there is some way to go before people who are self-funding routinely receive the help they need to make these difficult decisions (Melanie Henwood Associates, 2011).

Sarah found that an important aspect of her role was to advise and direct John and Mary to the services that would best meet their needs. She also acted as a central point of contact for John and for a number of agencies and individuals involved in looking after Mary. In this capacity she was able to iron out communication difficulties and ensure that the patchwork of care surrounding them did not start to unravel again.

It was inevitable that much of the detailed planning and negotiation in relation to Mary's needs took place between Sarah and John and involved Mary to a much more limited extent. John was therefore treated in some respects as a co-worker. Twigg and Atkin (1994) categorise social work with carers in terms of four models: the carer as a resource; the carer as a co-worker; the carer as a co-client and the superseded carer (whose caring role has been taken over by others). Tanner and Harris (2008, p.178) warn of the danger inherent in the 'co-worker' model of disempowering the client at the centre of the assessment. In this situation however, John was not simply a co-worker, he was also a resource, a client with needs in his own right and someone struggling to agree to others taking over aspects of his caring role. Sarah was very aware of the danger of excluding Mary, but she nevertheless found it difficult to include her in the process of planning her own care:

> I tried to involve Mary more, but it really wasn't possible for to engage with the decisions that needed to be made. I felt the best I could do was try to reassure her that I was someone she could trust – mostly through touch and gesture and listening to music with her. Also, they were such a strong unit that their needs were very much bound up together. I felt as confident as I could be that she would trust John to speak for both of them.

Liz Lloyd (2003) challenges the way in which social care services tend to categorise people as either 'service users' or 'carers', thereby promoting a narrow idea of carers as part of service provision. She argues instead for 'a relational approach that perceives caring as a normal activity in which we are all implicated in some way or another'. Drawing on the feminist ethic of care, Lloyd questions the rights based perspective by which social policy tends to concern itself with the individual rights of the carer and the individual rights of the client. She argues that policy should rather take account of interdependence and obligation and ways of fostering the caring relationship:

> It requires a shift of focus from relationships between carers as individuals on the one hand and service users as individuals on the other, to understand the caring relationship as the basis from which a range of responsibilities is negotiated, including responsibility to oneself. (Lloyd, 2003, p. 42)

It is of course important that social workers working with older people are aware of the potential for conflicts of interest between people in relationships which involve the giving and receiving of care. These conflicts can be extreme and require careful and empathic involvement from social workers and others. Furthermore the vulnerability of very frail older people and the potential inherent in caring relationships for exploitation and abuse is also real and demands vigilance and the capacity to make difficult and authoritative decisions.

In this case however, Sarah felt confident that by supporting John and Mary's loving and interdependent marriage, she was working in both of their interests. The relationship that Sarah was able to build with John helped her to understand his fear that his wife would be removed from his care. John in turn came to trust Sarah as a representative of the previously mistrusted 'social services' and to accept that she really did have an understanding of what was important to him and best for his wife.

Stephen A. Webb advocates a move away from the focus on what he calls 'caring actions' towards 'caring relations' in social work (Webb, 2006, p. 216). Others have similarly stressed the importance of a 'meaningful and constructive connection' (Trevithick, 2003, p. 168) or an 'emotional commitment' (Parton, 2003, p. 13). Such a commitment was evident throughout Sarah's work with John and Mary. While her 'actions' resulted in many practical improvements to their lives, her practice was rooted primarily in her caring relationship. Webb calls this

> the consistency of a fundamental orientation of goodwill towards those whom one works for and works with and towards the activities in which one engages. (ibid, pp. 220–221)

John's own attitude almost certainly helped Sarah to resist easy definitions of carer and cared for and to focus on the human relationship at the centre of this piece of practice. John hated being classified as a 'carer' and often reminded Sarah and other professionals involved in Mary's care, that he saw himself first and foremost as her husband. As Sarah came to know him better, John began to open up about Mary's past life and his own and to talk to her about some of the things that had been and continued to be important to them. Sarah recognised this as an important way in to her own relationship with Mary:

> He painted such a vivid picture of her as a district nurse, fighting and campaigning for her patients' rights, that I had this strong image of what she had been and in many ways, continued to be. Then there was their shared love of music, which seemed just as important to them both as it always had been.

Tom Kitwood, whose work Sarah describes as strongly influential on her practice, uses the concept of 'personhood' to encapsulate the idea of continuity of personality among people with dementia. Kitwood (1997, p.16) advocates the sensitive meeting of needs in a way that recognises the uniqueness of each individual and argues that professionals must find ways in to individual experience, including through the use of their own 'poetic imagination'.

Sarah was indeed able to engage imaginatively with John's portrayal of Mary's past life and therefore with the continuity between this and her current likes and dislikes. Her intimate understanding of Mary's 'individual biography' (Tanner and Harris, 2008, p. 141) informed the practical interventions that Sarah put in place and the ways in which she was able to advocate for Mary in her dealings with care staff, health professionals and others. She found for example that staff in the nursing home where Mary received day and respite care, were really interested in John's scrap book of cuttings about Mary's nursing career. The knowledge this gave them about Mary's past life helped to establish a link with her in the present as well as enabling John to share his pride in Mary's achievements. Also at Sarah's suggestion, the simple fact of Mary's deep and continuing pleasure in listening to music provided the care workers who visited her at home with a way of helping Mary to feel calm and safe by playing her favourite songs.

Sarah's practice in this situation was imaginative, inter-personally skilled, relationship gifted and humane (Howe, 2008). Like Rachel in the previous chapter, she succeeded in overcoming an initially fearful and hostile response and establishing a trusting and constructive relationship. Sarah would be the first to acknowledge that this involved a certain amount of luck – she and John and Mary clearly found it easy to like one another. However, Sarah managed to build on the warm connection she helped to establish to ensure that the support provided to John and Mary was effective and likely to continue to be so into the future.

5 Eric, Len and Nina: Growing Older with a Learning Disability

Questions to ask yourself as you read:

- In what ways might the needs of older people with learning difficulties differ from the needs of other older people?

- Is there a tension between adult safeguarding procedures and relationship based working?

- Why was time so important in this situation?

Eric, Len and Nina

Eric, an acting team manager in a rural community team for older adults, introduced the story of his work with Len and Nina, by saying that it *was* all about risk and thresholds of intervention. This is certainly a strong theme in what follows. However, as with all the narratives of social work done well, included in this book, it is also a story of the building of relationships of trust and care, which make other things possible.

When Eric first met Len and Nina they had been married for 40 years. They both had what he describes as a mild learning disability and had had occasional contact with specialist learning disability services. Nina was referred to Eric's team following the latest in a series of brief hospital admissions, usually following a fall at home. Staff on the ward were having difficulty communicating with Nina because of her speech impairment and felt that she needed a full assessment before she was discharged home.

The first time Eric met with Nina, it was on her own in the hospital:

It's quite difficult to follow what Nina is saying, but it isn't impossible. You need a bit of time to tune in and it helps to be somewhere quiet so you can really focus on her and reflect back what you think she's said, to make sure you've got it right. Anyway, she made it clear that she wanted me to talk to her and Len together, so I went back to do that the following day...

...As soon as I started to talk to the two of them together, I could see how they compensated for each other and had found ways to work together as a team. Len had a degree of speech impairment as well, but he was more able in many ways than Nina and could understand what was being said to him better. On the other hand, she was more organised and sort of made sure they stayed focussed on things.

In his first couple of meetings with Len and Nina, Eric found out that they had met through Len's sister when they were in their twenties and married a few years later. They had recognised their shared experience of living with a learning disability and had found ways of supporting each other:

Nina in particular would talk about meeting Len as if it was yesterday. She wouldn't have expressed it like this of course, but I felt that what she was saying was that it was a 'meeting of minds'.

Len had been a road sweeper all his adult life and had received a long service medal, of which he was very proud, when he eventually retired. Nina had cared for her mother for many years before her death and also worked part time as a cleaner in a local hospital. They were now in their late sixties and although Len was in good health, Nina was suffering from arthritis and had become quite frail. Len and Nina had no children and now had only intermittent contact with the remaining members of their families:

...so they were actually very much alone and very, very dependent on each other. Nina's movement had become pretty limited, so although they had held things together very well for many years, there was a danger that this additional challenge would make the difference between them coping and not coping.

Eric continued the process of working with Nina and Len and the other professionals involved to assess the support that Nina would need when she was ready to be discharged from hospital. At one point however, the assessment took an unexpected turn, which threatened to change the course of Eric's intervention:

> I received a phone call from the ward one afternoon to say that Nina had been discovered on the floor and had broken her wrist. Nina had told ward staff that Len had pushed her to the floor deliberately. This understandably generated a lot of anxiety and concern about whether Len was a danger to Nina.

As a senior social worker already involved in assessing Nina, Eric took on the role of gathering information and investigating what had happened. This was done within the context of his agency's formal procedure for safeguarding vulnerable adults:

> I was very glad indeed that I had already got to know Nina and Len quite well before this incident and that I had developed some skills in communicating with Nina in particular. I had to keep an open mind of course, but after some long conversations with both of them, it emerged that Len had been trying to help Nina to the bathroom. He had moved her awkwardly and she had fallen. She was angry and accused him of pushing her, without really realising the implications of what she was saying.

Eric was able to use the relationship of trust he had already built up with Len and Nina to establish what had really happened between them. If Nina's initial accusation had been accepted at face value or investigated by a worker with whom she had a less well-established relationship, the outcome might have been different. As it was, Eric made a clear professional judgement, informed by his knowledge and understanding of the couple and by the respectful and open minded discussions he had had with both of them. The completion of the Safeguarding investigation was not quite the end of the matter however. In spite of the result being accepted and recorded by the local authority and the hospital, Eric found that he had to

> do quite a lot of 'pouring oil on troubled water' to make sure everyone involved knew that Len was not in any way out to deliberately harm Nina.

Eric found himself advocating on behalf of Len in particular in order to ensure that none of the ward staff or others working with Len and Nina continued to feel suspicious of Len's motives towards his wife. At the same time, Eric was very conscious that Nina's fall had highlighted her vulnerability and the very real risks that she was facing as she became more physically frail:

I had no doubt that Len loved Nina and wanted to help her or that she wanted him to care for her, but she was very vulnerable and certainly likely to be at risk if we didn't make sure he knew when and how to help her to move safely and when to call for assistance from someone else.

The next stage of Eric's involvement was therefore to act as an intermediary between Len and Nina and the rehabilitation team who assessed Nina's needs at home. Neither Len nor Nina had been formally labelled as having a learning disability and did not have access to any additional support in this respect. However as a result of observing Len and Nina over a period of time and having established a relationship within which they felt comfortable and relaxed enough to share their fears and anxieties, Eric was able to ensure that additional support was put in place where necessary:

The hospital occupational therapist worked hard to get the flat adapted and equipment put in to make Nina as safe as possible. She and the physiotherapist also did a lot of work with both of them on how Len could help Nina to move around safely. It took longer – a lot longer for them to feel confident using things like the new shower or the hoist that had been provided than it would for most people. Sometimes they would say they understood when they didn't – it was a coping mechanism they'd always used and you could completely understand it. Anyway they were a bit more prepared to admit to me that they needed more help. Nina seemed to like my sense of humour and what started with laughter sometimes led to the sharing of important confidences.

Eric recognised Len and Nina's tendency sometimes not to admit that they didn't understand things because they were afraid of looking foolish or appearing not to be coping. Nina in particular talked of times when, as a child, her parents threatened to 'put her away' in an institution. As Eric came to know Nina better, he often used humour to put her at ease. This seemed to enable her to open up to him about her fear that if she and Len could not manage to look after themselves, they would not be 'allowed' to live independently.

By being consistently supportive and understanding of Len and Nina's situation and engaging imaginatively with their life experiences, Eric gained their confidence and trust. This enabled him to offer reassurance that it was okay not to understand something and to support them in asking for more help when they needed it.

As a result of the very full multiprofessional assessment that had taken place, extensive adaptations were made to Len and Nina's flat

49

and equipment was provided to help Nina to move around inside and outside the house. Once all of this was in place and Nina's wrist was sufficiently healed, she was discharged home with a minimal package of care.

In the two years since Nina's hospital admission, the couple have managed to remain independent, with only limited outside support. Eric organised some help from a local voluntary organisation to support Len and Nina in managing their finances and this continues. Apart from that, their main contact is with the local social services office where Eric works:

> They just pop in when there's a problem and either I or whoever is on duty helps them out. Neither of them can really make themselves understood on the phone and this really limits how much they can find out in any other way. I know it's not how the system is supposed to work – they don't really meet current thresholds for intervention, but it feels like genuine preventative work. In fact it has probably meant the difference between them being able to stay at home and be independent and the whole thing falling apart.

Eric tells of the time when a podiatrist told Nina she needed special shoes, which would take six weeks to make. Nina, believing she was not 'allowed' to leave the house wearing her old shoes, was preparing to stay indoors until the new shoes arrived. When Len came over to the social services office to see whether anyone could get the shoes made more quickly, Eric was able to phone the podiatrist who reassured Len that it was fine for Nina to go out in her old shoes while she was waiting for the new ones.

On another occasion Len and Nina received a letter telling them they had won a 'Euro lottery'. This was the sort of letter that most of us would immediately discard, but for Len and Nina it caused great uncertainty about whether they should telephone the number give to claim their 'prize'. Again Eric was able to explain that the letter was a scam and the importance of not responding to this sort of unsolicited mail.

> These were just two of many small interventions over the past couple of years. When they're not sure about something it causes great anxiety. In many ways Len and Nina are very capable and a great success story, but their vulnerability is real and they need ongoing support. There was another time when someone knocked on their door and tried to persuade them to spend thousands on building work they didn't need. They almost fell for it, but fortunately they checked with us before they signed anything.

At the time of writing, the rural office in which Eric is based is due to be closed. He and his colleagues will move to a town 15 miles away. He is currently trying to link Len and Nina to a range of voluntary organisations who will help to support them when they can no longer pop in to their local social services office:

> I worry about them. I worry that they won't quite meet anyone's threshold for a service. It's a pity because they ask for so little and yet the little we have provided over the last couple of years really has made a big difference in keeping them safe.

Discussion

Eric's work with Len and Nina was kind, empathetic and consistently respectful. It demonstrated a high level of imaginative engagement as well as the professional confidence to combine guidance and advice with consistent support for Len and Nina's own choices. Eric's focus throughout his work was on establishing a trusting relationship as a way of engaging authentically with Len and Nina's needs and wishes. One of the ways in which this was achieved was through a process of ongoing reflection on Eric's part about how he could best respond to an evolving situation. This was skilled practice which required time, creativity and careful use of self.

In their discussion of relationship-based approaches to practice, Wilson et al. (2011, p. 11) make the easily overlooked point that

> the professional encounter is unique to the professional and service user concerned and the relational dynamics are the combined result of their individual characteristics.

Alongside his professional experience and expertise, Eric brought his warmth, humour and outgoing personality to his relationship with Len and Nina. While this came naturally to him, Eric was also able to reflect consciously on the ways in which aspects of his character and personality contributed to the relationship. The insights that this engendered enabled him to use personal as well as professional dimensions of himself to demonstrate consistently supportive, relationship-based practice:

> I could tell quite early on that they felt comfortable with me – maybe because I could make Nina laugh. Anyway I had a way in and they seemed able to

confide in me. I knew the relationship I had with them was a privilege and something to be used carefully and responsibly if I was to help them.

As we have already noted, several writers have expressed their regret at the trend towards increasingly managerial or competency-based approaches to social work in recent years (Morrison, 2007; Jordan, 2001; Gregson and Holloway, 2005). One of the striking things about Eric's work with Len and Nina however was his imaginative engagement with their situation which was anything but managerial or procedural. Closely aligned to this was Eric's recognition that investing his time was essential to a successful outcome:

I spent a lot more time with them than I normally would. The safeguarding issue partly made that possible – it meant there was an additional process to go through and that gave me official permission to work more intensely with them. At the same time I don't think it would have worked if I hadn't. It was a complicated, fragile situation and if I hadn't been able to really get to know where they were coming from and understand their lives, I think the whole package could have fallen apart as soon as Nina left hospital. Then we'd have been back to square one – or maybe minus one.

Eric also recognised that the ability to enter imaginatively, yet accurately, into the thoughts, feelings, hopes and fears of another person is essential to effective relationship-based practice (Trevithick, 2003). As Nigel Parton (2003, p. 16) points out:

There is a range of skills, which have traditionally lain at the core of social work, particularly related to process and where the ability to negotiate and mediate with creativity are of particular relevance.

These were precisely the sorts of skills that Eric employed as he sought to understand the risks and the strengths inherent in Len and Nina's relationship. His awareness of the complexity and the fragility of the situation he was dealing with led him to focus on the process of getting to know and understand Len and Nina in order to help them make the most of their future lives.

The importance of seeking to achieve the outcomes that clients want has rightly been asserted as a priority by policy makers and practitioners in recent years (Glendinning et al., 2006; Bennett et al., 2009). Len and Nina, however, were not always able to be clear about what they wanted to achieve, nor were their goals static during the time that Eric was working with them. Rather, the solutions and strategies for keeping Nina and Len safe at home evolved over time through the process of their involvement with Eric and with other professionals.

Adams et al. (2009) liken social work practice to the performance of a musician engaged in the creative act of choosing in a planned way between myriad possibilities. This is not to suggest that Len and Nina's own choices and decisions were not central to Eric's work with them, rather that he resisted easy or simplistic interpretations and responded to new information as it emerged and as Nina and Len became more prepared to trust and confide in him. When Nina alleged that Len had pushed her over, Eric was able to stand back from the situation and reflect on his existing knowledge of Len and Nina's relationship in order to begin to draw out the truth. A more hurried or a less thoughtful approach, which took the situation at face value, could have had disastrous consequences.

Thoughtfulness and the confidence to use his extensive store of practice wisdom and experience to reflect on the situations he was dealing with were central components of Eric's approach. In common with many of the social workers we spoke to, Eric had a precise knowledge of agency procedures and statutory responsibilities and wove his practice expertly and confidently around these. Also like many other practitioners, his use of social work theories and methods was often unspecific and internalised rather than conscious or overt. Eric's practice was no less skilled for not being guided by an explicit body of theory however. As many social work commentators have argued, an ongoing process of reflection, which allows social workers to develop theory within a specific practice context, can allow them to work in ways which are highly 'situated' and responsive to a given situation (Fook, 2002; Wilson et al., 2011).

Eric reflected constantly on his growing understanding of Nina and Len's unique life experiences as they took him further into their confidence. This enabled him to alter and adjust his approach as he came to know them better. The changing context of Eric's practice, from an initial assessment in hospital to a safeguarding adults investigation, a complex process of rehabilitation and a period of ongoing support at home, added further to the complex and distinct nature of the work. Again, a reflective approach which enabled Eric to draw on his existing understanding of Len and Nina's circumstances and his long experience of difficult practice situations enabled him to fine-tune his response according to their needs.

Donald Schön (1987, p. xi) whose ideas have been particularly influential in the application of reflection to social work practice challenges the primacy of external sources of knowledge and highlights instead the importance of

> the competence and artistry already embedded in skilful practice – especially the reflection-in-action (the thinking what they are doing while they are doing it) – that practitioners sometimes bring to situations of uncertainty, uniqueness and conflict.

Similarly Jan Fook who suggests that for social work practitioners 'ways of knowing' can sometimes be a more helpful term than 'theory' argues that

> [y]our own interpretation will be made from your own subject position and may be made up of an amalgam of different types of ideas which come from your own personal history, formal theories you subscribe to, or your own practice wisdom. (Fook, 2002, p. 69)

Eric's practice demonstrated just this sort of reflection-in-action, working in combination with aspects of his own personality, knowledge, ideas and practice wisdom. This is clearly evident in the quote below where Eric describes Nina's words to him and his consequent insight into her vulnerability. It also demonstrates yet again the way in which Eric uses reflection within the context of what is fundamentally a relationship-based approach:

> *Nina said something like: 'of course you can't tell them you don't understand or they might tell you off or put you away somewhere – don't tell them I didn't know how to do it will you Eric?' – What I got from that was that Nina didn't see me as one of 'them' who might put her away or tell her off. It made me realise how important it was to keep a relationship of trust with her. It was the best possible way of keeping both of them safe. It really made me think ...*

Eric's awareness of Len and Nina's vulnerability and the potential for them to be misunderstood, overlooked or exploited was an important factor in the decisions he made about the best ways of working with them. Helping Len and Nina to have as much power and control as possible within their lives and to maintain the independencethey valued so much was central to Eric's practice. However, he also acted as an advocate and an adviser, often using the skilled insights gained through his relationship with them to interpret their fears and anxieties. On more than one occasion, Eric's gentle challenging enabled Len and Nina to admit to difficulties that might otherwise have gone unnoticed and unresolved thereby leaving them at greater risk.

Wilson et al. (2011) are among those who criticise the trend evident within recent social policy and manifested in social work practice towards treating clients as 'rational consumers, able to choose which services they want' (p. 7). They argue that this approach often fails to give consideration to the ways in which the personal and social circumstances faced by individuals impact on their capacity to make rational choices. This tendency to see people who are in need of support as 'consumers' or 'service users' in full control of their lives risks denying the existence of frailty and dependency which characterise the lives of many older people who use social work services.

Len and Nina were well able to make most decisions about their daily lives without help or interference from anyone else – they had lived independently for over 30 years after all. However, as they grew older and Nina in particular became increasingly frail, their vulnerability and consequent need for understanding, empathetic support increased. Without Eric's intervention, Len could have come to be seen primarily as a threat to Nina rather than a source of security and care. The equipment provided to help Nina move around at home could have gone unused because Nina feared to admit that she did not understand how it worked. Finally, without the ongoing, low-level support provided by Eric and the rest of his team after Nina was discharged from hospital, Len and Nina might well have been taken in by one of the financial scams or unscrupulous salesmen who sought to exploit them.

A simplistic interpretation of Len and Nina's right to make their own decisions based on the fact that they clearly had the capacity to do this perfectly well in almost every aspect of their daily lives could have left them vulnerable, isolated and anxious. As it was, Eric used his experience and his ability to practice reflectively and respond creatively to provide a series of meaningful and genuinely supportive interventions.

Part 2

Working Creatively in Organisations

6 Working Creatively in Organisations

Introduction

Perhaps one of the dangers of a book like this is that, in focusing on the human 'stories' of social work, the organisational constraints and frustrations within which these stories take place are underemphasised. As we have already said, the social workers we spoke to rarely mentioned policy or procedure or the mountains of paperwork they probably had to complete, but talked instead about their relationships with the people they were working with. So, having spent some time looking at the centrality of these relationships, we now want to examine in more detail the reality of working life and the organisational context in which they have to be built.

Most social workers are employed in statutory agencies, which, increasingly, involve partnerships with health professionals. These organisations are complex and frequently driven by conflicting political, financial and ideological imperatives. Traditionally, they remain bureaucratic structures, invariably with a 'command and control' style of management, with policies and procedures imposed from the top down rather than designed from the bottom up (Hughes and Wearing, 2007). Whilst individual teams may be very supportive environments, it can be hard for social workers to find their way around the organisation as a whole, or to understand where and how decisions are made. The overall organisational ethos may feel a very long way removed from the values of social work.

Each of the three case studies in this section illuminate aspects of creative organisational work and illustrate what it can look like in practice. In Chapter 7, the social worker, Maya, supports Bill to return home after an emergency placement. The following chapter tells the story of Stella, a woman who hides her dementia so well that no one notices it, and shows how her social worker, Trish, delicately negotiates the help that she needs at home. And finally, we look at Sinead, in Chapter 9, who supports Pauline after a stroke to set up her own assistance at home using a personal budget.

But, before moving on to the case studies, we will examine the organisational context a bit further and explore the characteristics of creative social work practice within it.

Managerialism and bureaucracy – Is it really that bad?

...the ways in which the social work role has been constrained by the organizational contexts... make it hard to assert that practice with older people is more than simply a treadmill of routinized assessments leading to unimaginative packages of care. (Lymbery, 2006)

On the basis of Lymbery's quote, you could be forgiven for thinking that social work with older people is very dull. The story of the relentless advance of 'managerialism' has been told so often that it has become something of a truism that social work with older adults is formulaic and routine, dominated by 'gatekeeping', risk assessment and tick-box forms. In this reductionist world, there is little or no room for 'traditional' social work values or for professional autonomy or judgement. All three of the social workers we heard about in the previous section were clearly worried that the kind of relationship-based work they described was under threat, and it was a concern that arose again and again in the discussions that we had.

It is true that there is an enormous amount of paper, or its electronic equivalent, and the sense of 'procedure overload' (Banks 2007, p. 5) will be very familiar to most social workers. Some of this has a positive purpose and, without any of it, the whole edifice of organised welfare would simply collapse. Standard rules help to make individual judgements more equitable; clients know what to expect when policies and processes are clear; procedures help social workers practise legally and the act of writing assessments or case notes is a way of reflecting on what has been said and deciding what needs to be done. Contracts and invoices may be dull but, without them, nothing happens. In the end, organising care for thousands of people is not an easy task and is bound to involve considerable administration.

However, other aspects of all this activity appear to have little benefit and may be positively counterproductive, wearing down both the social workers and the clients who are subjected to it. In practice, many of the processes around assessing both needs and finances are complex and unwieldy, taking up precious time and resources. In Chapter 17, Matt describes how he had to spend hours researching inappropriate placements in order to justify a more expensive, specialist placement to a meeting of senior managers, when he knew that a specialist placement was both needed and available. Indeed, some local authorities insist that all care packages have to be agreed at so-called panel meetings, which is a time-consuming and costly exercise. Even the basic building blocks of the community care process involve considerable repetition and duplication, as assessments, care plans and reviews are repeatedly completed by social work teams and, on different paperwork, by each service provider.

In large, bureaucratic organisations, forms and processes have a habit of taking on 'a symbolic significance beyond their functional value' (Hughes and Wearing, 2007, p. 36). One of the social workers we spoke to described how he could arrange transport for a client by email, but then had to fill out, by hand, a form to send to the relevant department, with a copy carefully filed away in a large ring binder. He had no idea what purpose this form served, but it always seemed quicker and easier to comply and fill it in. More seriously, where procedures are too prescriptive and detailed, they both take time (time that could be better spent in direct contact with the client) and encourage social workers to work in ways which, though technically correct, may become routine and unthinking. Having over-prescriptive forms and 'one-size-fits-all' guidance for Safeguarding Adults, for example, suggests that all Safeguarding referrals should be approached in the same way, whether the 'abuse' is physical violence by a carer who has come to the end of his or her tether, or systematic, deliberate neglect. However, in practice, labelling a stressed carer as an 'abuser' and the situation as one that needs to be 'investigated', if not done with extreme care, is both inhumane and very likely to make a bad situation worse.

As social work is by definition varied, there is also a tendency for organisational procedures to multiply in an attempt to cover every eventuality, becoming so long and unwieldy that they are impossible to use in practice. Munro (2011) highlights this as a major problem in child protection work and the same is increasingly true of social work with adults. In Munro's opinion, it is professional expertise within a broad policy and practice framework that needs to be developed, rather than the minute prescription of activity. Ferguson (2010, p. 1114) takes a similar line, arguing that 'elaborate bureaucratic routines... are manifestations of not only how individuals, but also organisations create defences against anxiety'. For individuals, following a process in the office may seem very much easier than dealing with the messy and risky reality on the ground. For organisations, the processes give a (probably illusory) sense of control and a basis for justification if things go wrong.

The related emphasis on targets and performance management has been particularly damaging to social work. Judging the work of an individual or team against standardised timescales and targets simply encourages people to shift their focus from helping the client to that of meeting the target. Social workers may feel, for example, that they have to spend time writing up each client visit as a formal review so that it can be 'counted' on the computer system as a piece of work in their name. Or, time may be spent documenting and inputting data for a Safeguarding referral when the situation itself is relatively straightforward, like a theft being dealt with by the police. There can also be pressure to open and close cases, so that a new referral, assessment or review can be added to the tally. As an unintended consequence, social work involvement becomes more repetitive and fragmented for clients who often have to go back to the beginning of the referral process, repeat their story and get to know someone different each time they 'come back' into the system. Even something going wrong (a care plan falling apart) may look like a success if it generates a review and adds to the number completed.

The 'systems thinking' occupational psychologist, John Seddon, argues convincingly that the only effective way of measuring the success of a service is for the people doing the work itself to define how it should be measured from the point of view of their clients or customers. Measures then become meaningful and, as they are 'owned' by frontline staff, there will be real motivation to make improvements based on the information collected (Seddon, 2008). By contrast, in the obsessive performance management culture of many social services departments, what is being measured is 'activity' because activity is easy to measure. This begs the question, is it the right activity as, in William Bruce Cameron's words:

> Not everything that can be counted counts, and not everything that counts can be counted. (Cameron, 1963 in Munro, 2011, p. 45)

Computerised care management systems are designed first and foremost to record formal processes and timescales and the reports that can be produced from this data reveal almost nothing of what is actually going on or how effective it really is. The social work itself is entirely hidden. As social work is not 'counted', many social workers feel that they should not really be doing it – that it is not something that their organisations value or want. Maya (Chapter 7) describes some directly supportive work she does with her client, Bill, and says:

It's beyond what we're supposed to do, but we do it, don't we?

And another, very experienced social worker we spoke to was even more explicit:

I long ago came to the conclusion that the best way to deal with senior managers is to tell them as little about what you are doing as possible. Just give them what they want to know to keep them away.

The truth is that the majority of senior managers would probably agree that a standardised response is not good enough, and are committed to providing a good quality service. But, like frontline staff, if they are judged by the number of targets they have met, or even if they perceive that this is how they are judged, it will inevitably influence and skew their priorities. For social workers, the upshot is that we often feel there are two quite different, and strangely disconnected, things going on within our organisations. At the bottom is our work with clients and, above that, a kind of parallel universe where detailed procedures are written, forms are created, information is gathered about timescales, numbers and dates, and reports are produced showing where the frontline has fallen short. What makes this all the more bizarre is that, although social work is not made visible or measured, it is not just an optional extra. Skilled and thoughtful work is key if local authorities are to fulfil their statutory obligations.

There are perhaps signs that this may be improving. Some local authorities have overhauled their processes and are reporting the benefits of, for example, simplifying the audit requirements for direct payments and the processes by which funding is approved (Carr, 2010). The Munro Review of Child Protection has, as we have said, done much to highlight the negative impact of a procedure- and target-driven system in children's services, calling for an end to 'nationally designed assessment forms, national performance indicators associated with assessment or nationally prescribed approaches to IT systems' (Munro, 2011, p. 10). There are experiments with social work practices and social enterprises, which aim to give frontline social workers more say in how their organisations are run. The government has explicitly said that it wants to reduce 'the data reporting and assessment burden upon councils' (Great Britain, Department of Health, 2011, p. 4). and, in measuring 'outcomes', more weight is being given to the client's own view of the service they have received.

So, there may be some light on the horizon, but even if it proves to be a false dawn, the fact is that social work with older people is far from dull. There clearly are major frustrations for social workers and a sense in which the 'real work' can easily be submerged under the weight of the bureaucratic demands placed upon it (Ferguson and Woodward, 2009). But, even so, a number of studies suggest that social workers actually have a relatively high level of job satisfaction, feeling motivated by the sense that they can and do make a difference to people's lives (Collins, 2008). A survey conducted in 2009 showed that social workers working with older people spent 25 per cent of their time in direct contact with clients and 72 per cent on client-related activities, including phone calls, joint working and case recording. Seventy per cent of those in adult services said that they were satisfied with their jobs (Baginsky et al., 2010). These figures may be far from ideal, but they do suggest that there is more to social work with older people than some people would have you believe. If you ask a practitioner what is wrong with social work today, they will almost certainly say the 'targets and bureaucracy', which are such a drain on their personal and professional resources. But, in our experience, if you ask them about an individual they have worked with, they will barely mention the paperwork. What is really going on within these managerial processes is incredibly varied and often very complex.

Creative social work

So, what does creative social work look like in the context of these large, often unwieldy, institutions? To practise well, social workers will always have to face two ways, on the one hand enacting the powers, duties and policies of their organisation whilst, on the other, focusing on the particular needs and circumstances of the person they are working with. We have, as it were, to be both personal and impersonal and just where we strike the balance between the two will shift, depending on the situation we are dealing with.

A personal, professional relationship

Social work has long understood that it is not enough just to want to help. 'Helping' always has a shadow side because the helper, particularly when they have an official position, holds considerable power and influence over the helped. Social workers do not provide help because they are kind (although they may be), but because their clients have a right to receive it and local authorities have a duty to provide it. So, part of the purpose of the structures and processes that we work within is to create a formal distance between us and our clients; a necessary objectivity in an entitlement-based, as opposed to a charitable welfare system:

> ... charity itself has the power to wound; pity can beget contempt; compassion can be intimately linked to inequality. To make compassion work, perhaps it was necessary to defuse sentiment, to deal coolly with others. (Sennett, 2003, p. 20)

And yet, as we have already discussed, there is a danger that organisational rules and processes create a real barrier between social worker and client, so that the essential sense of relationship is, at best, compromised and, at worst, lost. The system may be fairer, but it risks losing its humanity. As Arthur Frank puts it:

> Being responsible *for* can provide equitable delivery of services, but gone is the generosity that comes from feeling responsible *to*. (Frank, 2004, p. 126)

As we have already seen, research into clients' views of social workers repeatedly demonstrates that it is their personal qualities that are most valued – characteristics like 'committed', 'trustworthy', 'sympathetic', 'persistent', 'knowledgeable', 'warm', 'thoughtful' (Manthorpe et al., 2008; Beresford and Croft, 2004). The way in which social work is done is crucial and can transform standardised processes into a positive experience for a client. Of course, the type and extent of social work involvement vary from person to person. In the following three case studies, the work with Bill and Stella depended on their social workers establishing a strong and personal relationship. Pauline, by contrast, had close family and friends and what she principally needed was good advice and guidance. But, in order to provide this, her social worker still had to get to know her and to be sensitive and supportive in helping Pauline work out what her priorities were. It is interesting that, of all the social workers we spoke to most rarely used assessment forms as anything other than a framework to steer a conversation and help analyse and document the situation. Above all else, the best practice in social work organisations refuses to become impersonal, whatever the burden of paperwork.

Working with the system

However, it is an obvious if paradoxical point that the more social workers understand and the better they use the system in which they work, the more effective they are going to be on behalf of their clients. Going back to Matt who, as we mentioned above, had to seek senior management approval for the specialist placement, he was successful at least in part because he played by the rules, meticulously detailing the less expensive alternatives and demonstrating how each would fail to meet his client David's needs. Faced with this reasoned evidence, it would have been very difficult for his managers to turn his application down. Simple things, like using the language of eligibility criteria, law or policy when constructing a case, become second nature to skilled social workers. So, Trish, in Chapter 8, uses the principle of 'best interests' to justify additional support for Stella and, in Chapter 7, Maya argues that withdrawing Bill's service when he refuses to pay has both legal and resource implications.

More fundamentally, an equitable welfare system cannot exist without standardised guidelines to provide protection against the whims or prejudices of individual decision makers. So things like eligibility criteria and charging guidance (Great Britain, Department of Health, 2010a,b) are essential if resources are to be distributed fairly. This is what Olive Stevenson, in her perceptive analysis, calls 'the best of bureaucracy', the attempt to deliver 'proportional justice', or fairness across the whole system (Stevenson, 2004, p. 235). We may dislike the criteria themselves and believe that services should be free, but skilled organisational social work recognises the need for equity and does not simply ignore the rules.

Creative justice and discretion

Stevenson goes on to argue that, within this organised framework, there also needs to be a compassionate understanding of each individual situation, as a standardised system of equity can never allow for the myriad of different circumstances. This, she suggests, is a different sort of 'creative justice' – the ability to fine-tune the rules to a particular person. So, for example, in Chapter 7, Bill says that he does not need any help at home. He has the mental capacity to make that decision so, according to the principles of proportional justice, it would have been perfectly fair and defensible to have left him to it without providing any support. But Bill was deeply unhappy, self-neglecting and at risk of seriously harming himself and, from the perspective of creative justice, it would have been wrong simply to have taken him at his word and done nothing. It is in exercising creative justice that a social worker's discretion comes into play, the room to interpret the rules in the light of particular circumstances. As Evans and Harris (2004) point out, professional discretion is, in itself, neither a good nor a bad thing. However, if it is used well, it holds proportional and creative justice in tension. This is a theme which emerges particularly strongly in the social work with Bill and Stella, so we will be returning to it again later.

Critical pragmatism

What is, of course, debatable is the extent to which the system devised to administer proportional justice actually supports the use of creative justice and discretion, or whether the endless 'twisting, evading, bending and reinterpreting rules' (Webb, 2006, p. 2010) that social workers engage in is, by definition, a covert activity – a kind of 'guerrilla warfare' (Fergson and Woodward, 2009, p. 157). Working within the rules (as Stevenson herself points out) can certainly become very uncomfortable and even untenable if they are structured in such a way to be positively unjust. For example, we may well think that it is unjust that older people have to pay so much towards the cost of their care. Or local policies might state that, if no care home can be found at the local authority's standard rate, the authority will fund a more expensive placement, but only on a temporary basis until cheaper accommodation becomes available. Though technically 'fair', it cannot be 'just' to move a frail older person for a second time, when they are starting to settle into their new home and have already had the trauma of leaving their old one. Good social workers would muster every argument at their disposal to convince their managers that, in this particular instance, an exception should be made. But, there is no guarantee that they would succeed.

At a more fundamental level, there is widespread acknowledgement that the whole system for providing care to older people is 'unjust' in being chronically underfunded (Dilnot et al., 2011). A high proportion of home care workers receive little more than the minimum wage and many local authorities negotiate such low hourly rates that care agencies have to compromise the quality of care they provide in order to secure a contract (Equality and Human Rights Commission, 2011). The Director of Policy and Public Affairs for Age UK estimates that, on average, local authorities pay care homes £60 a week less per resident that the real cost of their placement. As a result, those funding their own care pay over the odds for their rooms, or homes insist that families pay a 'top-up', effectively subsidising the state. The support local authorities provide for younger people costs on average £78 a week, but just £53 for a older person (Harrop, 2011). The single most frustrating aspect of social work with older people is that even the most exemplary social work can be completely undone by poor quality services. And, what is more, these services may have been driven down in price (and quality) by the very local authority employing the social workers, who then spend more time and resources trying to put right whatever has gone wrong.

To add insult to injury, political rhetoric tends to adopt a relentlessly upbeat tone, removing itself so far from reality that it becomes positively misleading. So, for example, a local authority may say they are focusing on 'preventative work' whilst, at the same time, increasing the amount they charge for services. If, as a result, people decide they cannot afford the help they need, their situations are likely to descend into crisis, flying directly in the face of the preventative agenda. Or, whilst talking the talk of 'choice and control' and 'personalisation', a local authority may use the system of allocating funds for personal budgets to cut its expenditure, on the grounds that clients need to be 'creative' and 'flexible' in their support arrangements.

Confronted with these sorts of failings and contradictions, it becomes very tempting for social workers simply to put their heads in the sand or huddle under a 'blanket of weary cynicism' (Senior and Loades, 2008, p. 281). However, as social work, for the last four or five decades, has made strong claims about its commitment to improving unfair structures in society, cynicism (a negative acceptance of the status quo) is clearly not the answer. Instead, the best social work combines a fundamental pragmatism about what can be achieved in the here and now with a critical engagement with how things could be different in the future. The individual and collective challenge, as Maureen Eby says,

> ... is to find ways of ensuring that the ideas and aspirations are not totally lost whilst being utterly realistic about the constraints that exist in any organisational ... context. (2000, p. 118)

Faced with the enormity of what needs to improve, this may sometimes seem futile, but it remains central to the best practice. There is much which is open for debate, and social workers, who have so much direct experience of how the system affects the most vulnerable people in society, need to be a part of it. One of the social workers quoted in Ferguson and Woodward's book (2009, p. 75) puts it well when she says:

> If we don't take some sort of personal responsibility then we just become more insulated, more depressed and more demoralised and to me that's kind of what radical practice is, it's not allowing yourself to get demoralised and maintaining a sense of focus.

In *The Idea of Justice* (2009), the economist and philosopher Amartya Sen makes a distinction between two classical Sanskrit words, which both stand for 'justice', and are perhaps echoed in the ideas of proportional and creative justice we outlined above. The first, *niti*, refers to the abstract, institutional principles of justice whilst *naya* embraces the much more ambiguous, lived reality of people's lives. Instead of aiming for abstract perfection (which may simply serve as a distraction), he argues that we should instead ask ourselves whether we have made a particular situation less unjust:

> A theory of justice must have something to say about the choices that are actually on offer, and not just keep us engrossed in an imagined and implausible world of unbeatable magnificence. (Sen, 2009, p. 106)

Very often in social work the choices on offer are limited and sometimes the best choice is only a lesser evil. This is the reality and it is not defeatist to accept (or even to embrace) this and work with it. In some situations, it may simply be a question of seeing what we can do at this particular time to make this particular situation which involves these particular people less unjust. In others, the choices we have may include the real possibility of structural change where we can use our voices (and our votes) to press for policy or procedural reforms.

Conclusion

The following three case studies demonstrate how, in best practice, social workers negotiate the tensions of organisational working. They show that working creatively, especially as a statutory social worker, takes considerable thought, commitment and tenacity. You have, first and foremost, to focus on your clients as people and establish a personal, professional relationship. You need to work with the system, to know the policies and procedures of your organisation inside out, without letting them define what you do. Central to this is an understanding of creative justice and discretion, the close attention to the particular circumstances of the individual within an overall commitment to equity across the system. And, finally, you need to adopt a position of critical pragmatism, being realistic about what you can achieve whilst remaining critical, dogged and hopeful.

7 Maya and Bill: Balancing the Personal and the Professional

Questions to ask yourself as you read:

- Should social workers bend the rules for their clients?
- Why might the boundaries between personal and professional become blurred?
- Is self-neglect a 'lifestyle choice'?

Maya and Bill

It was Bill's general practitioner (GP) who contacted the Community Rehabilitation Service at the local hospital and asked them to visit him urgently. His general health had been deteriorating for a while and he now seemed to have given up. He was not eating, had had several falls, had stopped washing himself or using the toilet and his house was very cold. The team's remit was to try to prevent people going into hospital unnecessarily by providing them with short-term, intensive therapy at home to get them back on their feet again. But, after visiting Bill, they decided that he was unsafe to be at home on his own and, with his reluctant agreement, found him a temporary, National Health Service (NHS)-funded bed in a nursing home.

Maya was the social worker linked to the Rehabilitation Service and she met Bill a few days later. She soon realised how important it was to him to get home again as quickly as possible. Bill lived in a terraced house next to the railway track and had worked for the railways all his life. It was also opposite the municipal cemetery where his wife was buried. Every day he crossed the road to visit her grave and would sometimes sit there for several hours. A number of the falls he had had were when he walked across the road.

Bill had considerable insight into the reasons why he was no longer looking after himself. He saw no value in his life without his wife, but thought it was wrong to commit suicide. So, instead, he neglected himself:

> *He was in a low mood ... and we discussed whether he wanted to take his life, once I got to know him and could discuss that. And he said 'No I wouldn't ever do that'. He didn't think it was right to commit suicide. But he said 'The way I see it, I'm just going to continue smoking 50 cigarettes a day'. And the whole self-neglect was because he didn't really see any value in being on earth, but he didn't actually want to commit suicide. But in the way he was treating himself, he was slowly dying anyway.*

Bill had no family or friends so, whilst he was in a care home, the local authority had a duty to protect his property under Section 48 of the National Assistance Act 1948. Maya's first step was to use this legislation and ask Bill's permission to visit his house with the council representative responsible for 'Protection of Property'. It took two of them all day. The house was quite large and very cluttered, and it all had to be looked through and inventoried, with any valuables removed for safekeeping. In amongst everything, they found thousands of pounds in cash stashed away in different places, which Bill must have accumulated over a long period as some of it was no longer legal tender. The cash was taken away and paid into a ring-fenced account at the local authority for Bill.

As well as being cluttered, Bill's house was in a very poor state of repair. It was privately rented and he had an old-fashioned tenancy agreement, which gave him the right to remain there on a low rent. As a result, the landlord had done little, if anything, to make any improvements: there was no heating and it looked as if no maintenance had been done for years. It was also in desperate need of a clean. Rubbish had accumulated everywhere and the carpets were soaked in urine and faeces as Bill had struggled with incontinence and had tried to manage using a bucket.

Bill actually quite liked the care home, especially as there was a room where he could smoke, saying it was like a 'four star hotel'. But, he still wanted to get back to his familiar surroundings as soon as he could and would happily have gone straight away, returning to his house exactly as he had left it. There was no question about Bill's mental capacity to make this decision, but it was clear to Maya that she had to try to sort out the house first and ensure that Bill's situation did not descend into crisis again the moment he was home. An added complication was that, having found all the cash, Maya now knew that he was 'self-funding' and would have to pay the full cost of the care home, as well as any subsequent care arrangements. So she had the difficult task of trying to convince Bill that it would be better for him to stay in the nursing home for a few weeks whilst work was done on the house, even though he would have to pay for the privilege. If Bill had categorically refused, there would have been nothing legally that Maya could have done to keep him there, so a lot depended on the outcome.

Maya took a profoundly respectful approach in her negotiations with Bill, taking time to listen to and understand his perspective whilst being very honest and quite tough about her own opinions. She was aware that this would not have been right for everyone, but felt by then that she knew Bill well enough to know how best to talk to him:

> I think I worked out his character. You just have to be completely down the line with him... almost quite abrupt with him. There's some people you have to go round the houses, don't you? But I had to say, 'Look Bill, if you don't accept support, you're going to end up back in hospital. Do you want that? No. Right then... work with me'.... quite blunt and knowing that he would accept me being like that. Some people would think I was being rude. I think probably his wife was like that with him and when she went he had nobody to [tell him what to do]... So we're doing a bargaining – which we do quite a lot in our work, don't we?

However, though direct, Maya was also very sensitive in the way she proceeded, acutely aware of how difficult it was for Bill having changes made to his home in his absence. She had decided that the house needed a one-off clean and heating installed to make it safe enough, but she resisted the temptation to have it all cleared as she would have wanted it done. It would certainly have distressed him if changes had been made, which altered his sense of his house being 'home':

> When you think about it now, the trust he must have had in me to do that.... The way he chooses to live is up to him, but I cannot consciously discharge someone somewhere which is that unsafe.

There was pressure to get everything done as quickly as possible as Bill was paying a considerable amount for his room. But, Maya took great care to talk through the details with him and ensure that he had as much say as possible in all the decisions that were made. Over a number of visits, she built up a good relationship with him, established exactly what he was happy for her to do and ensured that he understood what was happening, especially in relation to what he would have to pay. Fortunately, Bill's memory was good, so he was able to give clear instructions and Maya made a detailed list with him of what she could remove and what he wanted left:

> His front room – he never went in there. I think since the day his wife died it was almost like his space where he spent time in there with her. So he did not want to have that room disturbed at all and refused to have that room cleaned. So that room was not touched.

Once Maya was sure what Bill was willing to have done, she was able to speak to the landlord, who agreed to install and pay for heating, and then arrange for a company to come and partially clear the house. It was very time-consuming, with Maya making frequent visits both to Bill and to the house in order to supervise the heating installation and the clear-up. Some of the money that had been found was used to pay for the cleaning and the rest was transferred into Bill's bank account.

> You have to be there to ensure that everything goes to plan. So, I spent a cold day, stood around watching people clear [Bill's] property.

The Rehabilitation Service had continued to work with Bill in the nursing home and their occupational therapist was very worried that he would not be safe using the stairs, persuading him to have a bed on the ground floor:

> He was adamant that he didn't want that. He wanted to go back to his bed upstairs. But begrudgingly he did agree to have a hospital bed put in there. So then I had to get his consent to us moving furniture out of there into the front room.

Maya did not disagree with the occupational therapist's assessment. However, she recognised that it was very much Bill's choice and took real pleasure in his stubborn assertion of autonomy:

> I don't think he slept in that bed once [laughing]! I think he went upstairs anyway into the bed that was full of woodworm!... You have to allow people to take those risks don't you?... That was his little bit of control. And I think 'great – good on you'.

After three weeks, Bill left the care home with the support of the Rehabilitation Service, who were able to help him on a short-term basis. His house was not transformed. The cleaners could not remove the carpet as the floor boards would have come up as well and it all still looked 'dark and dingy'. But it was at least basically clean and hygienic. Bill did not seem to notice any change. Nothing had been done that he had not agreed to and he settled back into his home.

Maya then worked closely with the therapists and rehabilitation workers to establish what sort of longer term help Bill would need and accept. Initially, he was so pleased to be home that he seemed quite motivated to do things for himself. But, as time went on, he stopped getting dressed, eating or taking his medication and his continence problems returned. Over the period she had known him, Maya had had several conversations with Bill about his depression and grief, as these seemed to be at the root of his problems. But, Bill was adamant he did not want to talk to anyone about it or try bereavement counselling or anti-depressants. The Rehabilitation Service was due to discharge him, and it was clear to them, and to Maya, that he was going to need ongoing support. So, Maya first referred him to the community matron, so that he had a health professional actively involved, and then started the next round of 'bargaining' with Bill about having care at home.

Once again, Bill was not keen and refused point blank when he realised he would have to pay for it. He had reasonable savings and Maya tried hard to persuade him that the time had come to spend these on himself, as no one else would benefit from them. As she put it to him:

> 'You've come to your rainy day, [Bill]. We are here … your rainy day has arrived. It's time to spend your money' was how I used to say it.

But Bill was adamant. He did not particularly want the care anyway, so why would he pay for it? This left Maya in a difficult position. She knew (and all the health professionals involved agreed) that without help at home, there was a very high risk that Bill's self-neglect would continue, his situation would rapidly deteriorate and he would once again have to be admitted to hospital or a care home, or would die at home through malnourishment and self-neglect. And yet, he was telling her that he would not have any help if he had to pay for it.

Thinking this through, Maya felt that there was a case for an exception to be made for Bill, because of the level of risk. Government guidance to local authorities about charging (Great Britain, Department of Health, 2012b) states that once someone has been assessed as needing a service, it should not be withdrawn because they refuse to pay for it (a fact not widely advertised). Different authorities may have varying policies in relation to this, but Maya knew about the guidance and used it to good effect.

In writing up her assessment, she stressed the likely consequences if care was not provided – both the human consequences and the impact that another crisis in Bill's situation would have on the department in terms of further work and resources. She was quite dismissive of her achievement in doing this:

> I don't know how I did that now – I must have just caught [my manager] at a weak moment! But I had serious concerns that, if we didn't provide a service for him, we could then be looking at potentially a death as a result of us saying 'OK, you've got the capital. Get on with it yourself.' I had to fight for him because I did not want that to be the consequence.

However, her arguments have a very sound logic which should make sense to a manager ultimately answerable for decisions about a client's welfare and responsible for the budget. At the same time, Maya recognised that there was an 'unfairness' in Bill being exempt from charges when other people, in the same financial circumstances, were having to pay. So, rather than simply accepting the decision to waive charges as being good for Bill, she continued to work with him to try to persuade him to contribute something. She repeatedly explained to him that one of the benefits he was receiving was given to him specifically to help him pay for any support he needed. Whilst he still refused to pay the full cost, he did eventually agree to pay an amount equivalent to that benefit towards the cost of his care.

The care plan that Maya agreed with Bill was for an agency to visit three times a day to help him with his personal care and try to encourage him to eat and drink enough. If Maya had been working strictly according to the local rules around eligibility, he should not have had help at lunchtime as he could have had a hot meal delivered more cheaply. But he refused this and she judged that he needed someone to come to try to make sure that he did eat. She made her decision 'fit' the criteria by fudging the issue on the care plan so that, on paper at least, it was principally a visit to help him with his personal care:

> I had to wangle [it and say it was] about changing incontinence pads – oh and while you're there could you prepare him a dinner please? But there were issues with his incontinence, so it was justified. ... though if he'd accepted community meals, that probably would have been sufficient.

Bill accepted and even seemed to appreciate the visits, though often would not let the support workers do much when they were there. He did not want to go anywhere or socialise, but Maya built some time into the arrangements so that, once a week, a support worker could accompany him across the road to visit his wife's grave.

With the care plan apparently settled, Maya was encouraged to close the case, but both she and Bill resisted this for some time. There always seemed to be something that needed doing – help paying bills or filling in a form. Or the community matron would ring and say that Bill was refusing the care and Maya would go over and talk to him again. On the way, she would do odd bits of shopping if there was something he needed.

It's beyond what we're supposed to do, but we do it, don't we?

Bill also frequently wavered about whether he would do better if he moved:

He'd ring me up and say 'I want to move into a care home ... I want to go, I don't want to stay here any more, I've had enough.' But then I'd go over there and by the end of the conversation, he'd talked himself back into staying.

Maya talked to him about an 'extra care' housing scheme in which he could have his own flat with a team of care staff on hand to provide help. Objectively, this would have been ideal for him and, on one occasion, he agreed. Maya secured a flat, but then Bill, once again, changed his mind. In the end, he could not bear to move away from the place where his wife was buried.

Eventually, Maya was told she had to close the case and hand it over to another worker to review it again in three months:

I didn't want to close him, to be honest. I really enjoyed working with him.

From an organisational perspective, the community matron was still involved and the care agency were providing a good safety net so that the risks to Bill were much reduced. Although she explained this to Bill, in practice he carried on ringing her to ask questions, and she carried on taking the calls, although she did not visit him again:

I don't think I would have got away with it – not in the age of electronic diaries. They know where you are!

Discussion

At the heart of Maya's work with Bill was a skilful and respectful balancing of the personal and the professional, 'mediating between the marginalised and the mainstream' (Davis and Garrett, 2003). Throughout her practice, she worked within organisational structures and processes whilst keeping her focus firmly on Bill as an individual. She became very fond of him and, although she had to challenge his perception of his situation, he came to trust her and clearly felt that she was someone he could talk to. Her assessment and care planning was very far from being a bureaucratic 'tick-box exercise'.

A research study into people's experience of palliative social work (Beresford et al., 2008) found that clients frequently used the word 'friend' when talking about their social worker. What was most appreciated was a warm, genuine relationship and flexibility in professional boundaries. However, although social workers may be perceived as being like a friend if they are helpful and understanding, it is always going to be a lopsided kind of relationship. In order to complete a good assessment, a social worker needs to be open and encourage the other person to talk, and they will not achieve this if they themselves are not genuinely 'present' within that conversation. But, at the same time, it is not a conversation between friends. As Richard Sennett says:

> To probe, the interviewer cannot be stonily impersonal; he or she has to give something of himself or herself in order to merit an open response. Yet the conversation lists in one direction; the point is not to talk the way friends do. (Sennett, 2003, p. 37)

Maya was very flexible in her work and genuinely cared about Bill, but it was a 'controlled emotional involvement' (Sheldon and Macdonald, 2009, p. 121) and she remained aware of her professional position:

> *If I no longer worked for the local authority, I would go and befriend him, make sure he's alright and do his weekly shopping. ... obviously I can't and I'd never blur that professional boundary ... I would have loved to have just popped in at the weekend if I were no longer a social worker.*

If a social worker did simply present themselves as 'a friend', they would be being dishonest with their client, pretending that it was an equal relationship. Maya, however, remained finely attuned to the dynamics of her relationship with Bill, always aware that she was in a position of influence. She did not shy away from giving him her views or her reasons for them, but she also constantly questioned herself, analysing her own thoughts and actions:

> He did accept [the support workers] coming in, but there was that sort of 'am I forcing it upon him' really... there was that grappling in my mind. Is it me wanting him to have this care more than him?

Charles and Butler (2003) suggest that this kind of critical reflection-in-action is perhaps the best defence against a mechanistic or routine response to a client. An uncritical reaction to the level of risk in Bill's situation might have been to steer him firmly towards a permanent placement where he would be safe and no trouble. Instead, Maya consciously engaged with the potential conflicts between Bill's safety and his autonomy, checking and questioning her own conclusions.

Maya also acted as an advocate for Bill within her organisation. Evans and Harris (2004) suggest that a proliferation of rules in bureaucracies actually increases the scope for social workers to exercise discretion within those rules, as the more detailed the rules, the more likely there are to be inconsistencies and ambiguities. So, in Bill's case, Maya 'wangled' a care visit at lunchtime so that a meal could be made for him. The rules stated that, if a hot meal was needed, the meal delivery service should be used. But, if someone needed help with something like using the commode, they could have a visit in the middle of the day. As the minimum time for a visit was 30 minutes, there would then be time to give the personal care and help could be given to make a meal. Did Bill need personal care help? It was all a bit borderline. Sometimes he did, sometimes he did not. Sometimes he accepted it, sometimes he did not. He did not quite fit the boxes. But Maya's judgement was that, overall, he needed the support of regular visits and was more likely to eat reasonably well if someone prepared the meal for him and chatted to him while he ate.

At the same time, she was not cavalier about the organisation's policies and, when Bill refused to pay for his care, she negotiated hard with him, understanding the need for equity between clients as well as the effects of his particular circumstances (a good example of the 'proportional' and 'creative' justice we discussed in Chapter 6). She used her knowledge of government guidance to argue for an exception to be made for Bill but, at the same time, managed to persuade him to pay at least something towards his care.

Maya's use of language illustrates well her ability to negotiate between Bill's individual life and her organisation, which had responsibilities towards hundreds of other people as well. Mary O'Hagan's account of her experiences in hospital (O'Hagan, 2000, p. 44) juxtaposes her own journal entries with the clinical notes that she later read, illustrating the power of 'official' language to define a person and their situation and effectively to silence the voice of the individual concerned. Whilst the psychiatrist interviewing her writes that she 'appears to be entering into a depressive phase. Withdrawn and quiet...not an easy patient to relate to', she is thinking 'he could see into every corner of my mind. I was afraid he had the power to trick me into letting out my biggest secrets. I was too terrified to talk to him'. It is a sobering reminder that the way social workers write about people carries tremendous weight; people's lives, for better or for worse, may actually depend on how they are represented by us.

When talking about Bill in her interview, the warmth of Maya's feelings towards him shone through, especially in her delight at his stubborn refusal to accept professional advice. This is the voice of daily conversation and relationship, the 'first voice' which Weick (2000, p. 399) describes as 'the essential voice of social work'. By contrast, when Maya read out what she had written about Bill, she had adopted the formal and dispassionate language of her organisation to secure the help that he needed:

> Mr Green does not feel that he needs support to meet his personal care needs. However, the concern is that if he does not wish to attend to these tasks, he will self-neglect as he was prior to admission to the care home. If he does not engage with services to prevent him from serious self-neglect... an adult protection case conference may need to be called.

This is the language of social services but emphatically not the essential voice of social work. We may wish that there was not such a gulf between the two, but the reality is that social workers have to use their organisation's language if they are to support their clients effectively. Maya's skill lay in being able to use the official discourse whilst not allowing herself to be absorbed into it or seduced into actually thinking in those terms.

All of this is not to say that there were no organisational restraints to hamper Maya's work with Bill. Although she resisted it for as long as she could, there was pressure on her to close the case once the basic practical care arrangements had been made, so that she could move on to work with other people. From an organisational perspective this may be the only realistic way to manage large caseloads. However, the effect is frequently a disjointed and unsatisfactory experience for the client, who may find themselves with a different social worker each time changes are needed to their care. Frustratingly, however good a piece of social work you feel you have done with a client, you often do not know how effective it has been. After Maya ended her work with Bill, the ongoing management and review of his care arrangements were handed to another part of the team and Maya had nothing more to do with him.

This fragmented way of working militates against long-term relationships with clients, making therapeutically supportive, as opposed to practical, social work considerably more difficult. Sheldon and Macdonald (2009) point to evidence that interventions with clear objectives and timescales are more likely to be effective than nebulous, long-term support and they warn social workers against the tendency to feel that they have to sort everything out. It is certainly true that social workers should not be a permanent presence in people's lives if they are not needed. In Bill's case, he had said he did not want any form of bereavement counselling, the risks to him had been reduced and the effects of his self-neglect ameliorated. So, you could argue that it was wholly appropriate to draw a line under the Maya's support, as time is limited and the public purse not bottomless.

However, there remains an uncomfortable sense that the underlying issue of Bill's grief was not (and could not be) addressed. If Maya had been able to continue, there was a chance that, over time, Bill would have opened up to her more, which might have led to a real change in his situation. This need not have been open-ended, unfocussed support, but could simply have meant that Maya, rather than someone else, continued to review Bill's care arrangements on a regular basis. Of course, it might not have made a difference as Bill might never have come to terms with the death of his wife. Maya eventually found out that, two years later, Bill had moved into a care home, although she did not know whether this move was planned by him or precipitated by a further crisis. And the disjointed nature of much care management meant that her organisation had no way of evaluating whether or not this could have been avoided.

Maya was very realistic about what she had been able to achieve. She hadn't radically transformed Bill's life or been able to help him work through the intense grief he felt at the loss of his wife. But, by building up a strong relationship and offering both practical and emotional support she knew she had made a difference:

> This was a guy who wouldn't let anyone through the door.... and I built up a really good relationship with him... and by the end of it, he still wasn't really accepting a support service. But, interestingly, he didn't just slam the door in their face. He let them in and actually I think he enjoyed the companionship and company... [and] I knew that there was someone keeping an eye on him.

81

8 Trish and Stella: Finding Creative Solutions

Questions to ask yourself as you read:

- In what ways do operational systems militate against good social work?
- Can social workers really change the system they work in or can they only find ways around it?
- How truthful should you be with someone with dementia?

Trish and Stella

Trish worked as a hospital social worker and first met Stella on the ward. She had been admitted after a fall and, from the information on the referral, it all appeared quite straightforward. Stella lived in her own flat without any help and had not had any contact with Social Services before. She was evidently an intelligent, self-sufficient person, had worked all her life in the civil service and had never married. Stella's hospital notes indicated that she simply had an injured knee and it looked as if she would only need a bit of short-term support at home whilst she recovered.

Stella disguised her memory loss so well that it had never been noticed. She had no close family and had gone about her daily life without anyone picking up on the fact that she wasn't managing:

> *Because she was such a bright lady, she covered it really well and...you would not know...and that was what had caught everybody out.*

Busy nurses on the ward did not spot any problem, even though Stella was faecally incontinent:

> *You know, she'd say to the nurse 'that's alright – I'll change my pad. I can sort myself out thanks'. The nurse – busy as heck – would say 'OK fine, I'll go off and do somebody else'. Actually she was in a real pickle.*

However, as Trish spoke to Stella, her dementia became more evident. She highlighted it with the nursing staff, who then took more time to encourage Stella to accept some help from them and started themselves to realise the extent of her memory loss.

Trish did not have very much to go on in assessing what practical help Stella would need once she was back at home. Stella herself simply said she would be fine and it was impossible to know how much she would be able to do for herself once she was back in a familiar environment. So, Trish initially arranged for her to have support on a short-term basis from the Reablement team, who could both help to get her physically back on her feet and, at the same time, try to work out what was really going on.

It took two or three weeks to understand the extent to which Stella was struggling, to build up trust and establish some routines, but little by little they made progress:

> It was a gentle, gentle, nudge, nudge, keeping [Reablement] at it and them feeding back to me.

Although there was no medical cause, she remained faecally incontinent. She had forgotten how to use the shower or taps as well as kitchen equipment like the microwave and toaster, so she was not eating properly and left food to go off in the fridge. Stella would have been horrified and humiliated if she had realised what she was doing. Even as it was, she was constantly apologising, saying 'I'm so sorry, I don't want to be any trouble'. So, both Trish and the support staff had to work with great sensitivity and tact to encourage her to accept help whilst not in any way undermining her self-respect or making her feel she had lost control of her life.

Some solutions were very simple. Stella was a tidy person and carefully folded up her soiled clothes and put them back in the chest-of-drawers. So, Trish bought her a laundry basket and it was then possible to establish a routine so that she put her clothes in the basket and support staff washed them. Other help was practical, like applying for money from a local charity and buying Stella a bed to replace the one that was badly soiled.

Once Stella had got used to having help at home and the Reablement team had established the kind of support she needed, Trish found a care agency to work with her on a long-term basis. This was not immediately successful. Trish had discussed with them the extent of Stella's memory loss, but the care workers were not as skilled as the

Reablement support workers and frequently took Stella at her word when said she had eaten or had had a wash. They would leave written instructions for her about how to use the toaster or microwave, but the notes did not make any sense to Stella:

> I found that very frustrating and disappointing. That... having written all this painstaking assessment and nobody reads the thing. And you think, you couldn't have put it any more clearly but you have to put it respectfully because it goes to the client.... Educating [the agency] was a whole piece of work in itself.

The other thing that became clear to Trish as she worked with Stella was that she had not been managing her paperwork and finances for some time. Trish started to support her with this and the more she did, the more she realised how little Stella understood:

> And then I got a feel for... I'm not quite sure how your finances are being managed here. What's going on? She clearly didn't know. She was paying an extortionate amount for a tiny little rental television.... and when I worked out the telly was worth about fifty quid and she had paid back about £900 for it, I was outraged.... But she didn't know any better.

It became clear to Trish that Stella did not have the mental capacity to make decisions about the overall management of her finances. So, she discussed the situation with the Finance Department and agreed that a potential way forward was for the local authority to apply to the Court of Protection to manage Stella's money for her. This would protect her and was, arguably, in her best interests.

However, Trish was also very aware that this would be taking an enormous amount of control away from Stella. Although she could not manage her finances as a whole, she was still very good at figures and arithmetic and she was perfectly able to pay for something in a shop with cash.

> When I thought about it, I remembered one of the things that she said was that one of the joys that she loved was to come up to [the local shops]. And she was physically mobile and I thought we're going from one extreme to the other here... there has got to be a middle way.... what can we do? what can we do? because it just felt so wrong.

Trish thought that the ideal would be to set things up so that enough money was held by the Finance Department to pay the basic bills, but the rest was paid into Stella's post office account so that she could still get money out and go up to the shops. However, when she checked this, the answer was an emphatic 'no, no that can't be done, that's not possible'. If they took on managing Stella's money, they had to control all of the funds.

Trish was not at all happy about this, but went back to talk to Stella about it:

> I was very honest with her... because she had sufficient cognition to understand. [I said] 'You seem to need a secretary or admin person to do your finances. We understand that, but the system is very clumsy. And it seems to be all or nothing.'... I'll never forget the way her face fell and when I went back and said to her that this is what we could do – we take the burden of running your home away from you. I could see that it wasn't really what she wanted.

Having seen Stella's reaction, Trish's frustration at the inflexibility of the system really begins to show:

> I mean... this is an independent woman... she had managed her life and then I come swanning in and say 'well you can't do your finances any more'. So I thought it through again and I thought, well OK, she can't get the money out, but she still wants money, so can she get access to her cash. I mean it's her flipping money for goodness sake.

Thinking it through again, with considerable tenacity, Trish realised that, although Stella wanted to be able to get her own money out of the post office, what was most important to her was that she had some cash so that she could walk to the shops and buy things for herself. Her solution was to argue for additional time in Stella's support plan for a care worker to collect some cash from the Finance Department each week and give it to her:

> So there was still a certain amount of autonomy there. She was no longer able to go to the post office, but at least she had a bit of dignity.

It was unusual for Social Services to pay for time to do this, but an exception was made as Trish argued that taking away all Stella's control over her finances would be more restrictive than necessary and would therefore not be in her best interests.

Stella now settled into a routine and was happy with the support she received. She was eating more regularly and accepting some prompting and help with having a shower and managing her personal care. She was still able to go up to the shops but had a system in place to pay her bills and protect her from financial scams.

As with Maya and Bill, Trish had to stop working with Stella once the arrangements were 'stable' and the ongoing management of her care transferred to one of the community-based teams. So again, frustratingly for her, Trish did not know how well the care plan had worked for Stella in the longer term and her organisation had no way of evaluating its success.

Discussion

Although the situations are very different, the way in which Trish approaches her work has much in common with Maya in the previous chapter. First and foremost, she takes time to build a trusting relationship – time which, as we discussed in Chapter 2, is fundamental to the best social work. In an organisational context 'taking time' is often viewed as something of a luxury – even indicating an inefficient way of working. We have already seen that statutory social services organisations largely measure (and therefore value) work with older people in terms of the number of assessments and care plans completed and the speed at which they are done. All of this creates the illusion that arranging support for older people is a straightforward business, which can be rationalised into a process, squeezing out the need for social work at all (Lymbery and Butler, 2004). Hospital social work, with its overwhelming emphasis on getting people out of hospital as quickly as possible, is even easier to caricature as little more than facilitating a speedy discharge.

However, the reality is that much 'care management' is very time-consuming and far from being a simple case of form-filling. Many older people's situations are complex and, as each is so different, social workers find themselves doing a whole variety of things as part of 'assessment and care planning', even if the paperwork they use is standardised. Maya had to count money, arrange a house-clearing, negotiate with a landlord and get heating installed as part of her 'care planning' for Bill. Trish had to apply to a charity for a bed, buy a laundry basket, pay bills and end a financial scam in her work with Stella. And both of them were involved in patient, sensitive and persistent work with their clients to establish what help they needed and how it could best be provided.

Like Maya, Trish had a sense that she was doing more than was required, or even wanted, by the organisation she worked for, but she still persisted in providing the support that she saw was needed.

And it was only by the grace of God that it was so nearby to my work that I could pop in once a week.

However, even though their work appeared to be unsupported and unrecognised by their agencies, the time they spent was actually intrinsic to those agencies fulfilling their statutory obligations effectively. The local authority had a duty to assess Stella. She had no family or friends, so the responsibility for facilitating her safe discharge, and everything that it involved, fell on Trish. If Trish had tried to assess Stella quickly by asking questions and filling in a form, she would have achieved little, as Stella would simply have said that she could manage. She might then have been discharged home with too little care, only to have some further crisis. Or, if a care agency had been introduced too soon and in such a way that Stella felt was intrusive, she might well have started to refuse help, again leading to further problems. Finding out about someone's finances (checking they are getting the right benefits and have systems in place for collecting their money and paying bills) is part of a thorough community care assessment. Once Trish had realised the extent of Stella's confusion about her money, it was her duty to follow this up within the Mental Capacity Act 2005 – legislation which requires a high degree of consultation with the client. So, quite apart from the human cost, working too quickly makes no organisational sense. Much better to spend the time at the beginning really trying to understand what is going on and introducing help gradually in a way that someone finds genuinely supportive. As Trish put it:

I mean you don't go rootling around in someone's cupboards on a first visit, do you? ...

Oliver James (2008) suggests that trying to assess people with dementia by asking them questions, quite apart from often providing inaccurate information, can be immensely distressing – something that should give us pause for thought when we consider how many questions doctors and social workers ask people with memory loss. The Alzheimer's Society agrees:

Asking questions puts a person with dementia under huge strain, causing them to search for recent factual information that they may not have.

> When a person with dementia continues to be questioned their well-being diminishes under the strain, and depression sets in to introduce further, unnecessary cognitive decline. (Alzheimers Society, 2010)

Trish's answer was to take a more conversational approach, 'not as an exercise in gathering *objective* data, but rather as a process of creative communication' (Jones and Powell, 2008). Her primary focus was to build a trusting relationship with Stella while she was still in hospital, finding out about her past and what was important to her. The objective facts about the help she needed would become clear over time.

Underlying this skilled work was empathy. Trish constantly checked and critiqued how she was thinking and acting by imagining what it felt like to be in Stella's situation. She had a very strong sense of (and admiration for) Stella as a proud, independent, single woman who had always managed her own life and was now fiercely hanging on to her dignity and autonomy:

> *She'd covered up [her incontinence] on the ward, which is quite something as you know there's a singular lack of privacy on those wards. To have managed to have not changed your underwear or pads for days and days and days is quite good going...*

and

> *I try and put myself in her shoes and see it from her perspective.... You know, [she's] been living her life, relatively isolated when suddenly she gets people stomping in and out of her home and telling her what to do.*

Trish talked about 'putting herself in Stella's shoes', a phrase which Sarah Banks uses in her discussion of empathy and moral perception – 'seeing the moral features of situations...noticing someone's discomfort, recognising their hopes, fears, resentments or pain' (Banks, 2007). Empathy itself, she argues, requires both involvement and detachment so that you can, at the same time, both feel for and think about the other person – the very qualities that we have argued are at the heart of good organisational practice.

Empathy is particularly important in working with people with dementia, helping them to hold on to their own sense of self and identity (Jones and Powell, 2008). And yet, if someone with dementia believes that they are managing fine, it is a delicate business trying to introduce help without forcing them to confront their memory loss and confusion. There is a real dilemma about how much to say and how truthful to be. If you say too little, are you denying someone control by not giving them the information they need? If you say too much, will you simply make them feel foolish or cause fear and distress by undermining their already fragile self-image?

> Telling the truth is clearly an important moral value, and telling the truth will always be the natural starting point. However, in circumstances where significant distress or anger is caused by verbally truthful answers to questions, because of the person's cognitive problems, then it may be more humane to find responses that evade or offer only a partial answer to the person's question, in order to minimise distress. (Nuffield Foundation on Bioethics, 2009, p. 105)

Trish shows considerable skill in walking this tightrope. Rather than trying to convince Stella not to put her soiled clothes back in the drawer, she quietly buys a laundry basket so that the new routine appears quite reasonable and normal to Stella. When talking to her about her capacity to manage her money, she avoids confronting her with the stark reality, but suggests that she needs a 'secretary or admin person' – again, perfectly 'normal' and the sort of help that many people need.

Trish's 'moral perception' also shows in the detailed attention she pays to Stella's particular circumstances. When thinking about the help Stella needed to manage her money, Trish refused to accept the standardised 'solution' to the problem because she knew that it would not be right for Stella. You could say that the Finance Department argued the case for a rather negative version of 'proportional justice' – that, in order to equitable, Stella would have to accept the same service as everyone else. However, Trish was concerned with 'creative justice', recognising the impact that taking away all control of her money would have on Stella. She did not talk explicitly about the Mental Capacity Act 2005 but had internalised, as an ethical issue, its requirement that any arrangements made in someone's best interests should be as unrestrictive as possible. So, she went back to the care arrangements and found another way of giving Stella some independence with her money, securing funds for additional support.

We have argued that social workers need to be both critical and pragmatic in order to work creatively in their organisations. There is a sense in which trying to be both 'critical' and 'pragmatic' is an impossible task, as pragmatism perhaps necessitates a degree of acceptance that being critical does not allow. However, the best social work docs embody both, even if it shifts between the two, sometimes more challenging and sometimes more accepting. Trish's work illustrates this well. When there were difficulties with the care agency, she refused to accept this as inevitable, but her approach to the problem was essentially a pragmatic one (railing against the inadequacies of social care provision at this stage was going to have little benefit for Stella). She worked closely with the agency on the ground, explaining to them what she had learned about Stella and trying to improve their understanding and response as much as possible. Similarly, she challenged the organisation's response to Stella's financial difficulties by coming up with a practical alternative. Like Maya, she argued why, in Stella's particular case, an exception should be made to the usual rules, so that time was allowed for a support worker to pick up some cash for her. Ironically, this change to the support plan would almost certainly have cost the local authority considerably more than a flexible deputyship arrangement would have done.

9 Sinead and Pauline: A Personal Budget

Questions to ask yourself as you read:

- What is the social worker's role when clients are managing their own care arrangements?
- How can operational systems support good social work?
- What should you think about when planning a multi-disciplinary meeting?

Sinead and Pauline

Sinead's work with Pauline is, in some ways, very different from the work described in the previous two chapters and gives an idea of the variety in social work with older people. Social services organisations inevitably standardise their systems and processes, partly simply to cope with the number of clients they are working with and partly to provide some basis for an equitable service. As we have been saying, one of the keys to creative social work is, as far as possible, to use these standardised processes as a framework without allowing the work itself to become routine; the processes have to be moulded to fit the people, not the other way round. With Bill and Stella, the process (assessment – care plan – financial assessment – review) was very much there in the background shaping the practice, but it was probably the actual work done rather than the formal processes themselves that mattered most to them. In Pauline's case, her support was arranged using a personal budget and the fact that she could take some control of the process itself was of real importance to her.

Like Trish, Sinead worked in an acute hospital and she first heard about Pauline at one of the regular ward meetings. Pauline was in her early seventies and had had a major stroke leaving her, initially, with impaired speech and very limited mobility. Up until then, she had been enjoying an active retirement in her village. She had been a teacher and was still a keen gardener and long-standing member of the Mothers Union at her local church. She also had a large family with children and grand-children living very nearby, so her house was full of people coming and going. She had never had any thought of needing help at home.

Sinead was attached to a particular ward in the hospital and attended weekly meetings with the doctors, nurses and therapists to discuss the needs of each patient. So, she was able to start talking to Pauline some time before she was ready to leave hospital, getting to know her and avoiding some of the intense time pressure which blights many hospital discharges. Pauline was, understandably, shocked by the sudden and devastating change in her health and circumstances and very anxious about how she was going to manage once she was out of hospital.

> ... she was really determined that she wanted to go back to where she lived before. She had quite a network of friends who lived locally and she'd literally lived there most of her life.

At the same time, Pauline was quite unrealistic about the amount of help she would need. She had, after all, never had any help of this kind before and believed that, once she was home, everything would come back to her again, provided friends and family rallied round and popped in from time to time. In reality, she needed help to get around indoors and outside and with washing, dressing and getting meals, as well as a lot of reassurance as she was very anxious about being alone. Members of her family were willing to help care for her, but they were not going to be able to do this on their own. So, in talking to Pauline about the future, Sinead had to steer a delicate course: she wanted to build up Pauline's confidence and wholly supported her wish to return home, but she also knew that its success would depend on Pauline accepting help from outside her immediate circle. She agreed with Pauline that they would arrange a meeting with her family and the medical staff on the ward to discuss the issues and make a plan for her discharge.

Multi-disciplinary discharge planning meetings can be daunting affairs and a number of studies have found that, whilst professionals may think that they have involved patients and carers in discussions, many people do not feel consulted (Social Care Institute for Excellence, 2005). Sinead made sure this did not happen by spending time with Pauline and her family before the meeting and then proactively supporting them in the discussions:

Often our role as a social worker is to try to make sure at these meetings this person is not lost… and that all the conversation and all the information is directed to the person and not to me, because we're talking about their care.

At the same time, it was important that Pauline heard the views of the professionals working with her, so that she was clear about what they were saying and able to make informed choices. Sinead viewed this not as telling Pauline what to do, but rather providing her with information and recommendations to consider so that she could come to her own conclusions. She wanted to encourage Pauline and build on her determination whilst, at the same time, questioning her conviction that she would be able to manage with minimal help:

So one of the things we were doing was not telling her 'well this is what's going to happen'. It was more 'this is what we recommend. What do you think about that?'… It was trying to, sort of, respect her views and her hope that she would get back home and, you know, be able to cope. But also respect that her family and friends themselves couldn't necessarily guarantee to be in so often. So we needed to support her and support them. So at that meeting [I was] trying to make sure that she didn't think we were all being really negative.

The meeting went well and a number of things were decided. Most importantly for Pauline, it was agreed that she would go straight home from hospital. In order to make this possible, Pauline compromised and said she would, at least initially, move her bed downstairs, which was for her a major change and a difficult decision.

She was able to sort of understand then – 'OK, well I know I want to be as independent as I can, but this is what the other people are saying about how things might be to start off with'. And I think it gave her a bit of understanding of why we were thinking that she needed some care to be going in.

Pauline's assessment (completed with input from therapists and nurses on the ward) indicated that she needed help with all aspects of daily living during the day and night. So, the local authority agreed to provide a personal budget equivalent to the cost of a placement in a care home. Planning how to use this money was then done jointly with Pauline, her family and Sinead:

We worked out a plan identifying what the risks might be if she were left alone, and Pauline and her family worked out who she could bring in to top up the support provided by the local authority. They worked out who they were going

93

to use and the costs around that. ... so they took on their own budget and from that budget worked out how they were going to spend it and called on their own informal support.

At the same time, Sinead completed a separate carer's assessment with two of Pauline's daughters, who were going to be most involved in caring for their mother. This gave them the opportunity, without Pauline there, to discuss any anxieties they had about their new caring role, making sure they knew about support available to carers locally and thinking about respite and contingency plans if they were not able to provide the care for a period of time.

They hadn't been carers beforehand, so we did an initial carer's assessment in the hospital and then at the 4 week review, we did another carer's assessment because they'd kind of seen a lot more of how it affected their day to day lives. That was the value really of having the carer's assessment and acknowledging the family's support. Even though you might sometimes be doing an assessment and have [the carer] there, I think actually doing a separate one can really show ... that you recognise the support that person gives.

Pauline was interested in employing her own personal assistants (PAs), but as recruiting PAs was going to take time, this could not be done before she was discharged. She could have moved into a care home on a temporary basis, but that might have made it more difficult for her to regain her independence. Pauline herself, understandably, hated the idea. So Sinead worked with her to break her aims down into stages; the first was to get home with the support she needed with basic daily living. Once this had been achieved, they could look at further community-based rehabilitation and how best to organise longer-term support so that she had as much independence as possible:

She went home initially with ... commissioned services and then converted that to a direct payment, so that they could have that time to find and employ the person they wanted rather than that being rushed.

To start with, her family stayed over at night and came in when the agency wasn't there. Then, as Pauline's confidence grew, she felt happier to be left on her own for some periods of time, using a pendant alarm to call for help if she needed it. She also started to accept that she did need support and to work out what was really important to her:

For her, she needed much more of the planning doing further down the line once she had really settled at home. Because it was actually quite difficult to get beyond the point [of her saying] 'I was fine before, I was fine before'.

Sinead helped to steer her through this process, understanding that it inevitably takes time for someone to adjust to such a traumatic change in their lives and encouraging Pauline to focus on one thing at a time:

If [someone] is at a moment of crisis actually pulling out from them what's important – sometimes, you know, you may not necessarily want to be talking about it at that particular point. ... It was like looking at Maslow's hierarchy of needs – you know, what are your physical needs and then, once we got to the 4-week review, going up a little bit further up those stages. Initially it was very much about getting washed and dressed, making sure you had someone to help you with feeding, you had your medication delivered, you had means to summon assistance if you needed it. It was looking at those aspects. And then when we got to the review stage, it was much more finding out about 'Well what things have you felt you have been missing?' – the social side – and working out how we were going to manage those.

By the four-week review, Pauline was sure she wanted to employ her own PAs. Although she had started to get used to the idea of having help, she hated having support workers in uniform or with badges, particularly if she was going out. She also wanted to be able to choose individuals for herself and feel in control of her own arrangements. She started to focus more on her life outside the immediate practicalities, building in time when she could have the assistance she needed to go to church or do her shopping.

With input from an employment support organisation, who were able to guide her through the complexities of payrolls, employment law, tax and national insurance, Pauline recruited her own PAs. Sinead set the payments up so that Pauline had some contingency money with which she and her daughters could arrange respite if they were unwell or needed a break, making sure that they had the necessary information and resources in advance:

It was trying to make sure that they did not have to come back to Social Services. ... that they had their own idea about how to [arrange] support. It gave them a bit more flexibility and control that they didn't have to come back and say 'I think we need a reassessment'. [The money] was added to their direct payment, so they could simply arrange it themselves. ... if they wanted to have respite or a bit of a break.

Sinead encouraged Pauline to think through her support plan in quite a lot of detail to make sure that it reflected what was important to her. This included things like how she liked her tea made and the kitchen left at the end of the day – details which may seem minor but only because they are the sort of things that many of us take for granted and have never had to spell out. This was all information that could be passed on to the PAs when they were employed, so that Pauline did not have give the same instructions again and again. Whilst Sinead physically wrote the plan, she checked with Pauline that it made sense to her:

[I would say,] 'This is what we wrote as the objectives... are they written in a way that you think is important?'... it's trying to make sure that you're not using jargon – making sure that the objectives are real objectives for the person.

Pauline was determined to be as independent as she could be and wanted to have as little paid support as possible. With further physiotherapy, she continued to recover from stroke and regain her confidence:

When we reviewed all the outcomes – feeling safe and supported at home, you get to see your friends – she felt that she was achieving all that.

Discussion

What struck us most listening to Sinead was the positive way in which she consciously and systematically used formal processes in planning Pauline's discharge. Whilst she did not describe it in terms of 'task-centred practice', she clearly took a pragmatic, problem-solving approach. Sinead's focus was to encourage Pauline to analyse her situation, taking into account not only her own views, but those of her family and the professionals involved. The difficulties she faced were then broken down into bite-size pieces and prioritised so that they could be tackled one at a time. Sinead was careful not to impose her own solutions, but gave Pauline time to find her own within the structures of the personal budget process.

However, in framing her practice around these structures, Sinead was not in any sense on a bureaucratic treadmill, following procedures for their own sake. At the discharge planning meeting, she was very aware of the danger of losing sight of the person within the process, and her focus was always on Pauline herself. Like all the social workers we spoke to, the 'assessment' was first and foremost a conversation (one that continued at Pauline's pace over a period of time), not a form-filling exercise.

> You need to have that rapport with a person so that you can have an open conversation rather than necessarily sit there with the form in front of you and go question by question... it can sometimes seem a bit of a barrier.

Sinead was also very aware that the approach she took would not necessarily be right for everyone:

> Sometimes it's important to have care planning meetings, bringing everyone together to talk and sometimes actually not, as that might be too much for the person, to get round a table and having all these people talking. So, it's about working out which way we should go.... It's about valuing the uniqueness of the person.

Sinead was attached to a particular ward and partnership working with her health colleagues seemed to be second nature to her – as it did to both Maya and Trish in their different, but still health-related, settings. Although ward staff and social workers may have different priorities when it comes to discharging a patient, Sinead appeared very confident in her role, arranging and steering the meeting and working closely with the nurses and therapists on the functional aspects of the assessment itself. Her partnership style of working extended to Pauline and her family as well, involving them every step of the way. She ensured that their views were listened to, but also exercised her prerogative, as part of that partnership, to share her own expertise and opinions about the help that Pauline needed.

We discussed in Chapter 6 how easy it is for social workers to become cynical in the face of constant change. Part of the difficulty is that there are often tensions and contradictions within the systems we work in. You can hear something of this as Sinead tries to communicate the positive, person-centred approach of personalisation without calling into question Pauline's eligibility:

> You want to write a plan that kind of best portrays how independent and well this person's doing. But actually on the flip side, you also have to say, well this is them on their worst day and this is why they need this level of funding. [And that can] come across as quite a negative thing about them.

But, Pauline's personal budget raises some other inconvenient questions. Ian Ferguson (2007, p. 388) describes the term 'personalisation' as one of the 'warm, persuasive words' whose connotations are 'overwhelmingly positive and...therefore very hard to be 'against' without sounding mean or curmudgeonly'. It is also a word that can mean very different, and sometimes contradictory, things to different people. On the one hand, it can be said to have its roots in radical service user movements, which have long campaigned for more active participation and control. On the other, it appeals to a market-orientated, libertarian vision of a society whose citizens take responsibility for their own lives and are able to purchase appropriate services from a range of options. Ferguson argues that, used in this way, the concept of 'personalisation' fails to acknowledge the enormous barriers of inequality, disadvantage and poverty that make 'active citizenship' so much more difficult. These are barriers that cannot be broken down simply by giving people more choice over their care arrangements.

Pauline was given an amount of money in her personal budget equivalent to the cost of a care home, but this was not enough to provide her with 24-hour care at home. Instead, she had to rely on her family to 'top-up' the support, by staying with her at night and providing additional cover during the day. This worked well for her, but would not be an option for someone without family or the financial resources to buy in private help – someone lacking 'social capital'. If the guiding principle behind personalisation is that of social justice (Duffy, 2011), it appears that, in practice, some will still be more equal than others (Lymbery and Postle, 2010; Ferguson, 2007).

Pauline was also someone who wanted, and was able, to be involved and to take control of her care arrangements, so chose to have a direct payment. How would 'personalisation' or 'self-directed support' be achieved for Bill or for Stella, so that they had as much autonomy in their daily lives as possible? To what extent was it actually achieved in the more conventional care arrangements their social workers set up with them? It seems unlikely that their priority would have been to receive a direct payment and manage their own care. If 'personalisation' is going to have a real impact, it needs to make meaningful improvements for people like Bill and Stella, as well as for those more obviously able to 'take control'.

Personalisation is also being introduced at a time when the government is focussed on cost-cutting in the public sector. Increasingly, local authorities are using a points-based system to calculate how much funding each person receives in their personal budget, making the allocation of funds highly centralised. Social workers could legitimately fear that, whilst there may be more flexibility in how money is spent, there is potentially much less room for professional judgement in how money is allocated. Is the motivation around the whole notion of choice simply market-driven – a way of driving down costs? Are concepts like self-directed assessment and the push towards direct payments simply a way of reducing the number of social workers and the amount of expensive, professional support? Do the failings of 'traditional' home care agencies mean that they are inherently resistant to the ideals of personalisation, or do they simply indicate that care workers are undervalued, poorly paid and have to rush from one client to the next? It may be relatively easy to find creative and less expensive ways of reducing a client's isolation, but how many creative and less expensive ways are there of helping someone to get up, washed and dressed every morning?

It is not difficult (and remains vital), to critique policy developments in this way. And yet, there is also a danger of throwing the baby out with the bathwater. Simon Duffy (2011) argues that government departments will always couch their policy documents in expansive and vague terms, so that they appeal to as broad a range of people as possible. In that they are trying to 'sell' change, it is not surprising that they avoid debate about the possible disadvantages of any policy. Leaving aside the question of whether policy should be developed and marketed in this way, the fact remains that, in amongst the aspirational rhetoric and conflicting agendas, there are ideas within 'personalisation' which do relate to fundamental questions of social justice. At its most basic, it advocates one of social work's core beliefs – that the aim of any intervention must be to give the client as much say and control as possible. Some of the 'tools' associated with personalisation, such as direct payments, person-centred planning or individual service funds, clearly aim to do this.

So, this is not something that social workers can wearily dismiss, but is something we need, where we can, both to use, and to argue about – to find ways of debating with local and national policy-makers what personalisation can and should mean to the people we are working with. Sinead's work demonstrates well how the best social work is not cynical about change, but uses new opportunities to very good effect.

Part 3

Difference and Disagreement

10 Difference and Disagreement

Introduction

The stories in this section all involve situations of difference, disagreement, tension or conflict. None of them include violent or threatening incidents of the sort that social workers working with older people are likely to face only rarely. Rather, they are the more subtle, everyday incidents that arise when long-standing tensions resurface or when relationships become strained by changed circumstances or differences of opinion. Sometimes differences are compounded by fear, misunderstanding or the fact that those involved simply do not know which way to turn. The social workers in the following three chapters respond to these challenging dynamics by demonstrating a wide range of skills and practice approaches, while the varied contexts and situations within which these episodes of practice are set raise a number of issues and topics for discussion. Some of these are themes that have emerged elsewhere in the book as characterising good practice in any circumstance, while others are specific to the stories that follow and relate particularly to work in circumstances characterised by difference and disagreement.

Working with difference and change

Social work with any client group can involve engagement with widely contrasting values, lifestyles and ways of being. Individual social workers regularly and inevitably encounter situations they find strange, unusual or personally difficult to deal with. Variations in class, ethnicity and gender contribute unavoidably to the experience of difference, as do many harder to classify ways of being that are unique to particular individuals and families. In work with older people, differences of age and generation, including the experience of ageing itself, can further challenge the expectations and assumptions of even the most skilled and well-intentioned social workers.

Working with difference and disagreement necessarily involves conflicting interpretations of the meaning of situations and how they should be understood and dealt with. In the chapters that follow, social workers are often shown working with families whose life-styles they find it difficult to fully understand and individuals whose choices they do not necessarily agree with. However, an under-standing shared by all three social workers in this section of the book, of the importance of not seeing themselves as 'the sole arbiter of the meaning of events' (Howe, 1994, p. 252), ensures that the client's own perspective is continually sought and valued. On occa-sion this is a perspective influenced by fear, defensiveness or misun-derstanding and skilled work is needed to agree on the best way forward. A willingness to work with people as they are, not with a pre-defined idea of how they ought to be in such situations, charac-terises the practice that is showcased here.

The changes that accompany older age can contribute to the tensions and disagreements that manifest themselves in some situations involving social work with older people. The very need for social work involve-ment in an older person's life suggests a physical or emotional need, which for some may be associated with new restrictions or losses and perhaps with an accompanying sense of frustration and anger. In other situations, social workers may need to be alert to the possibility of long-standing or unresolved past experiences having increasingly prob-lematic consequences for a person as he or she grows older (Ray et al., 2009). This is not to suggest that ageing is inevitably or even usually associated with struggle and difficulty, but in some situations it may be that long-standing emotional or practical issues become more acute as a person becomes frailer and more in need of support. On a very practical level for example, two of the older people in the chapters that follow are closely involved in the support of younger family members with mental health issues. In each case, as the older person's own growing needs reduce his or her ability to continue in the caring role, with all the anxiety that this provokes, a range of tensions emerge and skilled intervention is needed from the social workers involved.

Whatever the cause of the difficulties and life changes associated with older age, the stories in this section demonstrate the importance of valuing the strengths, expertise and life experience of older people as a way of working constructively with difference and disagreement. Bornat and Byetheway (2010) suggest that the current emphasis on eligibility criteria and working with only the most vulnerable may mean that social workers risk developing a biased view of older age and underestimating the resilience and capacity of older people. Certainly the tendency within adult social work to focus on the things that older people can't do means that social workers often fail to engage with the things they can do.

The argument has been made consistently in recent years that the relational aspects of social work with older people have been downplayed and devalued (Lymbery, 2005; Kemshall, 2002; Ray et al., 2009; Cree and Wallace, 2009). While most of us who are involved in work with older people would find this difficult to disagree with, the social workers we talked to consistently placed the relationship between themselves and those they were working with at the heart of their practice. As Clark and Lynch (2010) argue, the best way for social workers to support resilience in old age is through an inclusive, supportive relationship, which both acknowledges and focuses on the previous coping strategies of the older person. This necessarily involves engaging with the lived experience of the older person as central to what makes for who they are in the present (McDonald, 2010).

Engaging with ambiguity and unpredictability

Terry O'Sullivan (2011, p. 176), writing about assessment and decision making in social work, emphasises the unpredictable nature of the social world within which practice takes place:

> We live in a non-linear world of fluid relationships that form an open system where the future is uncertain and the present is often ambiguous.

We all know that people sometimes say or do things that are contradictory or hard to make sense of. We know that relationships shift and change and that sometimes, unexpected things happen. However, we are not always very good at acknowledging that this sort of ambiguity and uncertainty is part of the day-to-day reality of social work practice and can lead to unpredictable outcomes. It is not uncommon, for example, for help that has been asked for in a social work situation to later be refused, or for someone to simultaneously express a wish to be safe and choose to put themselves in danger. On other occasions people simply change their minds about what they want or need, requiring social workers to be flexible enough to move in a different direction or negotiate an alternative course of action. In some circumstances clients, family members and even professionals can interpret the same situation in different ways and reach widely differing conclusions about what needs to happen. Such 'multiple subjectivities' or 'competing truth claims' (Healy, 2005, p. 214) require social workers to be able to engage sympathetically, but purposefully with differences and disagreements. It is no wonder that Adams et al. (2009, p. 6) refer to social work as 'the complexity profession', and emphasise the need for practitioners to take account of 'the complexities and ambiguities that people face in real life'.

The uncertain and often unpredictable nature of practice can also mean that the outcomes of social work intervention are not completely positive or satisfactory for everyone involved. In situations of inherent conflict for example, it is likely that some areas of difference and disagreement will remain unresolved in spite of the best efforts of the social worker. It may be that an older person's long-standing emotional or psychological difficulties mean that tensions and areas of conflict continue even after the most skilled social work intervention. In other situations, irresolvable disagreement between family members may mean that 'one person's solution is another person's nightmare' (Adams, 2009, p. 20) and finding an outcome that will satisfy everyone remains impossible. It is important to remember however, that even where outcomes are not wholly successful the practice that takes place along the way may be very good indeed. Jones et al. (2008b) argue that social workers often demonstrate practice that is the best that could have been achieved in a particular time and place regardless of the final outcome. 'Best practice', they suggest, should therefore not be equated with a notion of 'ideal practice':

> Such a 'counsel of perfection' approach is not helpful either for users or providers of social work services, as it only adds to a view that the profession is constantly failing and the service delivered is never (quite) good enough (Jones et al., 2008b, p. 288)

This is not to suggest that outcomes are unimportant or that they should never be used as a way of measuring the impact of practice. Local authorities clearly have a responsibility to use public money wisely and to be accountable for the quality of the services they provide. However, the extensive criticism, referred to above, of the increasingly bureaucratic and procedural nature of social work with older people suggests that measurability of outcome may sometimes be valued more highly than an ability to work creatively and flexibly in difficult situations. The stories in the next three chapters all feature social workers who are working with complex issues of difference and disagreement. In each case, the process of the work itself evidently deserves to be judged as skilled and effective in its own right.

The current emphasis on fast 'through put' (Ray et al., 2009, p. 148) of assessments means that the ambiguity and uncertainty inherent in social work practice can easily be missed or ignored. Where the complexity of a situation is underestimated, tensions and differences are unlikely to be acknowledged and the overall assessment will therefore be less complete. It may or may not be possible or appropriate for social workers to intervene in difficult or long-standing family relationships or even in individual behaviour that others find problematic. What is important though is that social workers seek to 'take account of and respond to the complexities and ambiguities that people face in real life' (Adams et al., 2009, p. 6) in ways that enable them to work effectively in difficult situations. The social workers in the following chapters respond to a variety of challenging circumstances in different ways depending on their particular personalities and approaches. What they share, however, is an ability to reflect critically and creatively on their work and to resist the domination of their practice by prescribed or procedural ways of working. Nigel Parton (2003) suggests that characterising social work as art rather than science is one way in which notions of ambiguity and unpredictability can be accommodated in practice. Adams et al. (2009, p. 7) make a similar point when they compare social workers to musicians whose every performance is unique and whose practice involves choosing 'in a planned way between myriad possibilities'. They go on to link the idea of social work as a creative act which requires engagement with complexity, to the concept of 'thoughtfulness', which 'is or should be, the six-sevenths of the iceberg of practice lying below the surface of visible actions' (Adams et al., 2009, p. 7). The importance of a critically reflective, thoughtful and creative approach to practice, however this is expressed, resonates strongly with the practice that is demonstrated in this and indeed in other sections of the book.

The challenge of working with risk

You can read a lot more about the skills and challenges of working with risk and the safeguarding of vulnerable older people in the final section of this book. However, the notion of risk is also strongly implicated in the situations of tension and disagreement that arise in all three of the following chapters. This is to be expected given the increasingly central position of risk within social work assessment. Circumstances where older people are perceived to be putting themselves or others in danger are often highly emotive and can lead to differences of opinion about levels acceptable of risk. At the same time, the process of identifying and responding to risk, while supporting the rights and autonomy of older people, means that social workers often find themselves in the midst of conflicting values and responsibilities that cannot be resolved without a high level of skill and professional confidence (Tanner and Harris, 2008).

Sometimes tensions, disagreements and conflicts can be anticipated in situations of risk, although they may be no less challenging for that. In circumstances where accusations of abuse or neglect are central to an intervention, for example, social workers will expect to deal with high emotions and feelings of anger and distress. Similarly in situations where older people lack the capacity to make choices about risk, social workers will find themselves using mental capacity or mental health legislation to protect their clients from harm or danger. However carefully and skilfully such decisions are negotiated and communicated, they will sometimes predictably generate anger and conflict, requiring the use of 'sensitive authority' (Douglass, 2005, p. 42) and a range of other highly skilled responses on the part of the social worker.

In other social work contexts, risk may be associated with difference and disagreement in more complex and unpredictable ways. The extent of the emphasis on risk in social work is itself a matter of concern to some commentators, who suggest that unreflective risk assessment can amplify difficulties and tensions rather than resolving them. Bornat and Byetheway (2010, p. 1119) are among those who argue that social work 'has become enmeshed in the identification and codification of risk factors' in increasingly routinised and prescriptive ways. The danger is that an over-emphasis on risk and particularly on averting risk taking is likely to reinforce taken-for-granted ideas of older people as passive and dependent (Thompson, 2006). Ageist assumptions are deeply embedded in society and older people are often assumed to be particularly vulnerable and in need of protection from harm. While the responsibility to protect may be an overriding concern in some situations, an uncritical approach to risk is likely to lead to inaccurate assumptions about older people's needs. This can, in turn, lead to defensive forms of social work that Cree and Wallace (2009, p. 53) argue are 'uncongenial to the development of human qualities likely to promote engagement in discussion of what counts as good practice in social work'.

An over-reliance on risk assessment tools and procedures in work with older people threatens to promote an idea of social work as subject to prescribed interventions and predictable outcomes. As discussed above however, the ambiguity and uncertainty of practice mean that predictability is more often than not a misguided assumption. Cree and Wallace (2009, p. 51) make the point succinctly when they assert that 'the one certainty in social work that does exist is that there are no certainties, at best probabilities'. The importance of assessing and re-assessing risk, with an awareness of the unpredictability of the outcome, is in fact essential to the safety and well-being of older people. As Terry O'Sullivan argues, it would be naïve and dangerous to believe in the existence of a wholly reliable risk assessment tool or procedure that could

> accurately assess the level and likelihood of a danger occurring, and the danger of the social world we live in means that it is unlikely there ever will be (O'Sullivan, 2011, p. 176)

Most of the social workers we talked to emphasised the centrality of risk in their work with older people. While some used formal procedures and assessment tools more flexibly and creatively than others, they were all conscious of an agency expectation that social work intervention would be framed in terms of risk assessment and risk management. The striking thing about the practice described in this section and elsewhere in the book however is the way in which it resists the over simplification of risk and does not base decisions on taken-for-granted assumptions about the needs of older people. Judy, whose work with Dorothy is the subject of Chapter 13, was not the only social worker to talk about the complexity and uncertainty of working with risk and the particular challenges that arise in situations of difference and disagreement:

> There was clearly a high risk that Dorothy would have another fall if she went home, but it was a near certainty that she would get really depressed if she stayed in the nursing home. I felt she had the capacity to make the decision, but not everyone agreed with me – capacity assessment isn't an exact science and neither is risk assessment. I wish they were.

Judy's practice, like that of the other social workers in the next few chapters, exemplifies the assertion by O'Sullivan (2011) that analysis and intuition are compatible and complementary and that both are crucial to decision making. This is social work that recognises the potential for risk taking to be a positive activity, while also being real-istic about both the uncertainty of outcomes and the reality of frailty and vulnerability. Furthermore it is social work that involves reflection on different perspectives and an ability to use agency tools and proce-dures flexibly in the context of professional judgement rather than as an end in themselves.

Multi-professional working

Work with professionals from disciplines other than social work is an important component of the stories in this section of the book, even where the main focus of the narrative is on the relationship between the social worker and the client. As Barrett and Keeping (2005, p. 21) point out, 'the complexities of health and social care are such that service users' needs are unlikely to be met by professionals working in isola-tion'. All of the social workers we talked to were collaborating in some way with other professionals in the community, hospital or residential or nursing homes. At its best multi-professional working is creative and complementary, resulting in a better and more comprehensive service to the client than a single individual or professional group could provide. It is also the case that multi-professional relationships can themselves be a source of difference and disagreement. For example, when Judy whose words are quoted above, says that not everyone agreed with her judge-ment about Dorothy's ability to make her own decision, she is referring to the district nurse, with whom she was working closely. Loxley (1997, p. 1) talks about conflict being 'interwoven within interprofessional collaboration' and it is certainly the case that different professions do not always share the same perspective or priorities for intervention. The tendency for each group to use its own specific language and profes-sional jargon (Barrett and Keeping, 2005) can compound these dispari-ties, just as open discussion and careful role negotiation (Cook et al., 2001) can help to overcome them.

Judy did not succeed in reaching agreement about Dorothy's needs with the district nurse, but they did find a way of working together in Dorothy's best interests, while their differences ensured that the process of decision making on Judy's part was particularly thorough:

> We were both concerned about what was best for Dorothy, so we did man-age to continue to work together. I think her disagreement meant that I really looked at the situation from every angle and kept asking myself whether we were doing the right thing.

Like other social workers in the following chapters, Judy was able to acknowledge the complexity of the situation she was working with and think beyond the boundaries of her own professional perspective. Robert Adams (2009) suggests that social workers often occupy a unique position on the boundary between different people and diverse views of their situations. While most other practitioners work within professional territory that is clearly designated, he argues that 'social workers draw on a variety of disciplines and have the capacity to work across many different kinds of boundaries' (Adams, 2009, p. 32). This is not to suggest that the contribution of social work is superior to that of other professions, rather that it can be more difficult for social workers to define their particular contribution within multi-professional groups. The ability to work creatively with complexity and contradiction and to span the boundaries between people and perspectives offers a helpful way of understanding the social work role.

Working with strengths and solutions

Individual social work practitioners will each have their own approaches to dealing with tension, difference and disagreement. It is to be hoped however that as reflective, reflexive individuals, they all bring their unique knowledge, experience and practice wisdom to bear in difficult or conflictual situations. Nevertheless there are recurring, interconnected themes in the three chapters that follow. The importance of drawing on people's strengths and capacity as a way of moving through and beyond difference and disagreement comes up again and again. Linked to this is a consistent emphasis on the future and finding solutions or ways forward for individuals at the centre of difficult situations.

The formula for strengths-based practice is summarised by one of its main proponents in the following terms:

> Mobilize clients' strengths (talent, knowledge, capacities) in the service of achieving their goals and visions and the client will have a better quality of life on their terms (Saleeby, 2006, p. 1).

Saleeby himself points out that while this recipe may sound uncomplicated, the work that follows from it is not necessarily straightforward or easy. One of the challenges is that service provision in health and social care too often centres on the things that people can't do rather than those they can. This focus on deficit, usually constructed in terms of risk, characterises a social care context within which Karen Healy (2005, p. 151) attributes the growing popularity of the strengths perspective to

> its emphasis on respect and service user self determination. The strengths perspective emphasises optimism and creativity, and in doing so, offers an alternative to increasingly defensive and risk-averse practices that have become commonplace as a result of the growing influence of the dominant discourses.

For social workers to move beyond risk-averse practice in order to focus on the strengths of an older person in this way demands a good deal of personal and professional confidence. The social workers we spoke to sometimes found that the process of enabling older people to assert their rights and choices contributed to the differences and disagreements they encountered. This was particularly likely to be the case when other professionals or family members took a very traditional or protective view of how older people should be treated. As experienced practitioners however, the social workers were able to analyse and justify their methodology and decision making with confidence and clarity. In all three cases the social workers' thoughtful determination to affirm the strengths and resources of those with whom they were working ultimately helped to resolve or at least to find ways forward in difficult situations.

Social work that values strengths and self-determination and seeks to move away from blaming or locating the problem within the individual inevitably involves optimistic, future-oriented ways of working. Terry O'Sullivan (2011, p. 6) uses the term 'solution building' to describe the sort of solution-focussed capacity building practice that is likely to emerge from strengths-orientated social work. Of course, social work with older people sometimes means working with those who are close to the end of their lives and it might be argued that future-oriented approaches have limited relevance in such situations. However, the practice demonstrated in this and other parts of the book suggests the opposite – that the imperative to identify priority issues for older people and find positive, empowering solutions that will address them is strongest of all for those who do not have long time to live.

In situations of disagreement and difference, a solution-focussed approach offers the potential for enabling those involved to use their strengths and resources to seek ways forward rather than remaining entangled in past disagreements. As you will see in the chapters that follow, this can involve social workers as mediators or advocates, helping to facilitate communication and resolution between individuals in conflict. Malcolm Payne (2012, p. 52), writing about what he calls 'citizenship social work', advocates a solution-oriented approach and suggests that social workers can act as 'cultural translators' between older people and their families or other parts of the community. He points out that

> [m]any people have not thought how the different life experiences of their older relatives gives them varying cultural expectations in life and, therefore, preferences. Alternatively they view the likely preferences of their relatives through the lens of their own experience.

The concept of 'cultural translator' resonates with the idea of social workers as 'boundary spanners' (Adams, 2009) discussed above. Social workers with an ability to reflect critically on different perspectives and to engage imaginatively with the feelings and experiences of others are uniquely well placed to be able to mediate and seek resolution in situations of difference and disagreement.

Conclusion

The practice demonstrated by Sue, Judy and Fiona in the next three chapters illustrates the range of every day issues, conflicts and dilemmas facing social workers and their older clients. The experience of difference and change is an inevitable part of growing older and is therefore of fundamental concern to social workers. Most older people will experience some loss of friends, family and familiar others as well as changes in physical functioning and the range of activities available to them. Shifting roles and responsibilities within families also have the potential for old tensions to re-surface and new differences to emerge. The skill of the social workers in the following chapters is to acknowledge and work with change and difference rather than seeking to ignore or to work round it.

Closely aligned to the above is the ability to engage with ambiguity and unpredictability. People in stressful, life-changing situations do not always behave sensibly and rationally, nor are solutions always clear or obvious. The ability of the social worker to reflect critically and thoughtfully on the behaviour of others and on their own decision-making processes, emerges again and again as a key characteristic of tolerant, effective and enabling practice.

Risk is another central theme in social work with older people and is explored in detail in the final section of the book. However, making sound judgements about the assessment and management or promotion of risk and risk taking are also recurring themes in situations of difference and disagreement as will be seen in the next three chapters. The use of relational skills and professional judgement in ways that avoid both taken-for-granted assumptions about older people and an over-reliance on risk assessment tools ensures that the social workers' decisions about risk are holistic and individualised.

Multi-professional working emerges as another important theme in this section. Sometimes effective collaboration between social workers and other professionals is revealed as the key to resolving differences. Elsewhere, perceptions about levels of acceptable risk or priorities for intervention create disagreements between professionals. In such situations a commitment to seeking agreement in order to provide the best care and support to the older person at the centre of the intervention is needed from everyone involved. It may be however that social workers, with their broad social perspective and practiced ability to appreciate different viewpoints, are able to span professional boundaries in ways that are particularly helpful for everyone involved.

Finally, each of the social work interventions in the following chapters is broadly strengths-based and solution-focussed. The social workers involved avoid defensive, risk-averse practice in favour of future-oriented approaches that explicitly value the contribution of the service user. The techniques and methods used in working with difference and disagreement involve negotiation, compromise and sometimes the authoritative assertion of professional judgement. They require the social workers to be reflexive about the impact of their involvement, alert and responsive to people's feelings and able to make thoughtful, reflective decisions with an awareness of the complexity of their work.

The practice demonstrated here is not 'perfect' in every respect, but all three social workers show an impressive awareness of the seriousness and the delicacy of the interventions in which they are involved. Situations that involve tensions or disagreements are particularly challenging and demanding. As you will see however, they also offer opportunities for social workers to make a uniquely valuable contribution to the resolution of differences and the promotion of positive change.

11 Sue and Alice: Working with Complex Family Dynamics

Questions to ask yourself as you read:

- How might family roles and responsibilities change as an older person becomes more dependent?

- Is there a limit to how far social workers should respect people's lifestyle choices?

- What social work skills are needed to balance competing needs and perspectives within a family?

Sue and Alice

Alice, an 87-year-old African Caribbean woman, lived with her grandson and his wife in a two-bedroom ground floor flat, owned by the local authority. Several other members of Alice's large extended family lived nearby. In fact, it was another of Alice's grandchildren who telephoned the local social services office to report angrily that Alice was not 'being properly looked after'.

The case was allocated to Sue, an experienced social worker in a locality team, specialising in work with older and disabled adults. Looking back on this initial referral, Sue talked about the importance of keeping an 'open mind' when visiting a family for the first time:

I got a strong steer – a very strong steer from the granddaughter who made the referral. She told me in no uncertain terms how things were. She was obviously concerned and I respected that, but you can't go into a new situation with a list of assumptions about what's going on. You have to hear what the people who are most involved have to say before you can make any kind of assessment.

Sue's involvement began with a visit to the family at home. There she met Alice, her 35-year-old grandson Michael and his wife Ellen. It was immediately apparent to Sue that Alice was in need of a lot of help and support. She had very limited mobility and had clearly experienced some cognitive damage as a result of a recent stroke. Alice herself appeared unkempt and her clothes were obviously dirty. It was also quickly evident that the relationship between Alice, Michael, and Ellen was complex and unusual. In spite of Alice's physical disability and marked confusion, Michael and Ellen seemed to look to her as the decision maker in the household, while Alice herself, spoke often of needing to 'look after Michael'.

Sue began to explore the roles taken by different members of the family. At the same time, she took care to respect the right to privacy of everyone involved and to remain aware of her responsibility to listen to each individual's interpretation of his or her situation:

> It's important not to assume you have the right to know everything about the way people organise their lives. Unless there are immediate, overriding issues of abuse or harm, you have to earn the right to people's confidence.

The picture that emerged from Sue's initial assessment visit was complex. She found a household characterised by periods of intense conflict and dispute, but also by reciprocal expressions of care and concern and a high level of mutual dependency. Alice had been and in many respects, continued to be, a powerful personality whose position at the head of a large extended family seemed to be fully accepted by her many children and grandchildren. For years, Alice's role had included helping to look after vulnerable family members and she regarded her grandson Michael as being in particular need of her care and protection. Michael's white Irish wife Ellen seemed to be somewhat excluded by the wider family, but appeared to have a close relationship with Alice and for some time had been the person most involved in her intimate care.

Michael and Ellen were both vulnerable in their own right. Neither had a diagnosis of learning disability, but both seemed to need significant help in managing their daily lives. Ellen had a strong tendency to overeat and at the point of Sue's initial involvement, her weight had recently increased to a debilitating 32 stone. This meant that Ellen was struggling to manage her own personal care and could now do very little to support Alice. Michael had been dependent on his grandmother to help and direct him in most aspects of daily living. Until Alice herself became physically frail, this had included putting out clothes for Michael to wear each day and tying his shoe laces for him.

Sue described a delicate equilibrium that had established itself in the household. For some years, Alice had needed a relatively small amount of help with personal care and domestic tasks. This was something that Michael and Ellen had been able and willing to offer. Throughout this period Alice had remained very much in charge and had been able to advise and support Michael and Ellen in managing their finances and organising the household. She had also played a vital role in helping them to resolve the frequent conflicts in their own volatile relationship. This was an arrangement which suited everyone and seemed to be underpinned by a strong sense of loyalty between the three of them.

As Alice's health deteriorated and her short-term memory began to fail, she came to require an increasing amount of care and help herself. Ellen had continued to work full-time, but Michael had given up his job in a local abattoir to 'look after' his grandmother. It was evident that this arrangement represented a significant reversal of roles and one that everyone in the household was struggling with in their different ways.

Sue found Michael difficult to engage during her visit:

> He wasn't unwelcoming or hostile, but he was constantly restless and distracted. Although he said that he was his grandmother's 'main carer', he didn't seem to feel that her specific physical and emotional needs were anything to do with him.

Ellen, by contrast, was always willing to chat to Sue:

> She was more able to describe the problems in the household, but Ellen also had a particular take on how things were. On one level, she was happy to accept that Alice might now need more support than Michael could give, but she also struggled to see Alice as someone who was vulnerable and at risk. She knew that Alice wasn't eating very well and that her clothes were soiled and dirty, but her attitude tended to be that everything would be ok or that things would be sorted out tomorrow or the next day.

Alice herself sometimes joined in the conversation and was sometimes inevitably excluded from it. Sue therefore had to take particular care to ensure that Alice's perspective was at the centre of her assessment:

> I tried hard to include Alice in the family discussion, but she was really quite confused and kept coming back to Michael and what he needed. It was

important for me to spend some time talking to Alice on her own – that enabled her to focus more on her experience of the family situation and what she wanted. It was absolutely clear that she saw herself at the centre of this big family and that she wanted to remain at home for as long as possible. At the same time she was very vulnerable and really not very aware of her own vulnerability.

With Alice's permission, Sue was able to gain information and advice from her general practitioner (GP) and from hospital staff who knew Alice as the result of a brief hospital admission some months earlier. Sue also spoke to several members of the extended family, who she described as

very willing to offer an opinion about Alice's care, but reluctant to give any regular support.

Sue's assessment was thorough and detailed. However, even with a range of professional contributions and close discussion with Alice and her family, she still needed to balance a range of competing and contra-dictory perspectives. In order to ensure that the family members were supported effectively, Sue had to see beyond both the angry accusa-tions of Alice's granddaughter and Ellen's easy-going assessment that everything was fine. It was important for her to challenge Michael's role as 'carer' – one which he readily embraced, yet seemed unable to carry out in practice and Alice's account of Michael as the one who needed looking after.

You have to work with people where they are, not with some idea of where or how they ought to be. This family was in difficulty, but that wasn't surprising – the roles in the household had been turned upside down. Michael was struggling to cope. He wanted to look after his grandmother, which was a great starting point, especially as it wasn't a family where men tended to see themselves as carers. But he and Ellen could barely look after themselves and Alice was finding it dif-ficult to accept that she couldn't do the things she used to without help. Michael loved his gran, but he was well outside his comfort zone. He just didn't know what he was meant to be doing and he was taking quite a bit of flack from his brothers and cousins who didn't think it was a man's job to be a carer.

This was a situation which required understanding and the building of a supportive relationship, but also a confident, independent profes-sional judgment on Sue's part:

I didn't feel that Alice was in immediate danger of serious harm or that she needed to be rescued, but things had to change... I was quite clear with everyone about that. There was nothing malicious or deliberately neglectful about the care that Michael was providing, but it definitely fell short of keeping Alice either safe or comfortable.

Sue communicated the outcome of her assessment to Ellen, Michael and Alice. She made it clear exactly why she believed that Alice needed additional help in a number of areas if she were to remain safe and well. In order to agree a way forward, Sue needed to respect what was 'normal' for this family. Ellen and Michael's understanding of Alice's needs was not the same as Sue's. However, by listening carefully to each family member and building on their strengths and abilities, a care plan was agreed, which incorporated support for Michael in his role as carer, as well as a realistic recognition of his need for time to himself.

At the heart of the package of care which Sue negotiated with Michael, Ellen and Alice was a daily visit from a care agency to help Alice get washed and dressed safely. This went well for three weeks, during which time everyone involved reported a noticeable improvement in Alice's well-being. Then Ellen telephoned the social services office to say that the family could look after Alice by themselves and no longer needed outside help. Sue realised that Ellen's call coincided with the arrival of a letter informing Alice about the contribution she would be expected to make from her pension and benefits towards the cost of her care. Although Sue had fully explained the process of means testing to the family, she was not surprised that the full implications had only been taken on board by Michael and Ellen when they were faced with an immanent reduction in their income.

Sue could have interpreted Michael and Ellen's refusal of services on financial grounds simply as exploitation of Alice. However, she had seen and heard enough of the way in which the family worked to understand that they were only just holding things together physically, emotionally and financially. The means-tested contribution may have been reasonable in terms of objective, standard criteria, but Sue understood that the disorganised lifestyle of this family meant that it was beyond what they could manage to pay.

Alice's pension and benefits had always formed part of the general household income, although she still insisted on giving Michael weekly 'pocket money' and believed that giving generous presents to her great grandchildren was an important expression of her role. Ellen and Michael had catalogue debts which they hardly admitted to themselves and almost certainly did not disclose during the financial assessment. A simple means test is unlikely ever to capture this sort of complexity, yet the degree of financial planning which would have enabled the money to be found for Alice's care was beyond Ellen, Michael or Alice.

Michael and Ellen seemed increasingly to be closing the door to all outside help and fears for Alice's safety were growing. The strong relationships Sue had established meant that she was one of very few health or social care professionals that the family were willing to talk to. However, before Sue's next planned visit could take place, the situation in the household broke down; Alice contracted a urinary infection and was admitted to hospital.

This time several more members of the wider family became involved and Sue found herself having to negotiate a high level of conflict and disagreement about what should happen next. In spite of several carefully planned meetings, she struggled to achieve a consensus within the family about how best to meet Alice's needs when she left hospital. Alice herself was now experiencing acute memory problems. She no longer had the capacity to make a clear judgement about her own future, but was nevertheless continuing to indicate to Sue her strong preference for returning home. Finally an agreement was reached that Alice should go to a residential home for a few weeks of respite care. As Sue recalls:

> Everyone needed some breathing space, including me! Alice wanted to return home eventually and there were services we could put in as well as offers of help from the wider family, which made me believe it could be done. But there were also long-standing feuds and resentments and huge differences of opinion about what was best for Alice. Sometimes I felt a bit out of my depth. As a white worker in this big, loud, mostly black family, I struggled to get my professional perspective across.

Throughout the course of her work with the family, Sue recognised that the particular challenges of the situation meant that the pace of her work had to be driven by their needs rather than agency requirements:

> There were timescales and procedures, as there have to be in any case, but I did need more time than usual to build strong relationships in order to make sure Alice could go home and be safe. I had to work at their pace. Fortunately my manager recognised that and supported me. In the end there were savings for the agency because Alice was able to be at home for longer and of course, it was what she and most of her family wanted.

Sue continued to work closely with Ellen and Michael and, with other family members to prepare for Alice's return home. In order to seek solutions and find a way forward for all three of them, Sue had to explore the difficulties they were facing with honesty, openness and respect:

> Ellen and Michael did let me in and told me a lot. I reached a point where I felt I had permission to be very honest and to challenge them about the impact of their lifestyle on them and on Alice. They didn't always agree with me, but they knew I understood how things had got to where they were. I think they knew I was basically on their side.

Sue also worked closely with the residential home where Alice was staying for respite care. Together, they were able to help Alice become more accepting of personal care from people outside her immediate family, while continuing to involve Ellen and Michael closely in preparations for Alice's return home. Sue also spent time directly supporting Ellen and Michael with practical and administrative tasks such as letter writing and the payment of bills. She was able to put them in touch with people who could help them to help themselves including a debt advice agency, a slimming group and a black carers group.

A care package was negotiated, which involved a high level of personal care for Alice, regular attendance at a day centre, a meal delivery service and a clear set of tasks which Michael agreed to carry out. This time, there was no argument about the requirement to pay for Alice's care, rather, there was an honest discussion about how the family finances could be organised in order to make this possible.

Alice remained at home with Ellen and Michael for a further six months. During this time, there were significant small successes as well as familiar difficulties. With more help from another family member, Michael and Ellen began to get their debts under control. This enabled them to buy new clothes for Alice whose physical well-being had improved considerably as the result of a healthier and more regular diet. For a while at least, Michael and Ellen's own relationship also seemed less volatile and the atmosphere at home became calmer. Sue kept in occasional touch with the family during this period as well as talking to care workers who were visiting regularly, in order to monitor the situation:

> Everyone was making a big effort. Ellen and Michael really did want Alice at home and she wanted to be there; they did the best they could to make it ok for her. There were still arguments and they all drank a lot, but there was a routine and some sort of shared agreement about the importance of prioritising Alice's needs. Eventually Alice's condition deteriorated and she had to go

121

*into a nursing home, but actually by then it was the right time for everyone –
including Alice.*

Discussion

Social work is a complicated, challenging and highly skilled activity.
The sometimes messy reality of people's lives means that the context
within which practice takes place can be hard to pin down, difficult
to understand and sometimes dauntingly unlike anything encountered
before. Social workers may find that the complex situations through
which they are required to navigate are subject to differing and
conflicting interpretations by those involved. A perspective of imaginative, empathic engagement, which seeks to work creatively with
difference and build on strengths and capacity, can offer a positive way
forward as Sue showed in this situation.

Listening to her talking about her work with Alice, Ellen and Michael,
it was clear that Sue found this a puzzling and sometimes frustrating
household to work with. At the same time she was clearly aware of the
need to suspend some of her own assumptions in order to work with
this family as they were, not as she or others might have expected them
to be. This resistance to easy or taken-for-granted assumptions about
individuals and the relationships between them reflects Anne Brechin's
definition of 'critical' practice as 'open minded, reflective appraisal that
takes account of different perspectives, experiences and assumptions'
(2000, p. 26). Sue's practice was sufficiently responsive and flexible for
her to be able to 'situate' it (Fook, 2002, p. 40) within the specific and
unusual context of the household, without feeling thrown by family
dynamics that were outside her usual expectations or experience.

In addition to the unusual and sometimes disconcerting levels of
interdependence within the family, Sue had to negotiate a number
of different views of the situation she was working with. Ellen and
Michael's perception of Alice's needs was not the same as Sue's, while
Alice's own interpretation was different again. Furthermore other
members of the extended family asserted a still wider range of ideas
about what the issues were and what should happen next. In order to
make sense of so many different and conflicting ways of understanding
the situation, Sue had to work respectfully and responsively with
those involved, while moving towards her own reasoned professional
judgement. It was clearly not possible for Sue to harmonise all of the
perspectives she encountered, however a series of conversations based
on what Hugman (2003, p. 1031) calls 'a negotiated accommodation

of perceptions' helped her to find enough common ground to be able to work constructively with the family.

Terry O'Sullivan (2011, p. 83) talks about 'practice wisdom' or 'practical wisdom' as

> [t]he capacity for reflective judgement that involves the ability to make or support sound decisions based on deep understandings in conditions of uncertainty.

Sue did not try to over-simplify the situation in which she was working, nor did she attempt to resolve all the conflictual or problematic elements of the relationships she encountered. Instead she used her practice wisdom to negotiate the way forward in the context of complex and changing family dynamics.

The relationships between Michael, Ellen and Alice were characterised by a powerful mutual dependency. While this often generated intense conflict between the three of them, it also united them, sometimes in disagreement with their extended family. Sue recognised both the strengths and the difficulties engendered by Michael, Ellen and Alice's reliance on one another. In this respect, her practice resonated with 'systems' approaches which advocate the importance of working with complex relationships in the family and in wider society (Healy, 2005). Alice's increased dependency and her transition from 'carer' to 'cared for' represented a significant change in the family system. The fact that Alice's sense of herself as a carer continued to be a powerful part of her identity, while Michael did not stop needing and depending on his grandmother, meant that Sue was working within a particularly intricate network of interdependency.

Adult social care services in the UK tend to construct those with whom they work as either 'service users' or 'carers'. Liz Lloyd (2003) highlights the dangers of such a narrow conceptualisation. Instead she advocates a relational approach which works with the family as a 'whole system', stressing diversity, reciprocity and interdependence within networks of care. Part of Sue's skill in this situation was to recognise that meeting Alice's needs and ensuring her safety necessarily involved direct, creative and relational work with Michael and Ellen as part of a reciprocal family system.

In this family as in many socially and economically deprived households, the intricate relationships holding individuals together were financial as well as emotional. While financial abuse is a real and present issue for many vulnerable older people, the rights and wrongs of what belongs to whom should not be over-simplified. Sue might have interpreted Ellen and Michael's wish to discontinue the service that Alice was receiving, as a straightforward attempt to control Alice's money for their own purposes. On an immediate or surface level, this might have been an appropriate response. However, Sue's understanding of the complex and interdependent nature of the family system meant that she was able to situate Ellen and Michael's actions within the context of their lives and relationships. This engagement with 'individual biography' (Adams, 2002) enabled Sue to adopt a more nuanced and critically aware course of action which helped to resolve the situation rather than apportioning blame.

Practising with an awareness of context, as Sue did in this situation, required a high level of critical professional judgement. She recognised that the complexity of the family's situation was unlikely to be captured by a standardised assessment of Alice as a client or of Michael and Ellen as carers. Sue also resisted either seeing herself as 'the sole arbiter of the meaning of events' (Howe, 1994, p. 525) or accepting uncritically any one family member's interpretation of the situation. She was generous, empathetic and supportive in her approach, but at the same time a thorough, realistic and critical assessment of Alice's needs enabled Sue to make a clear professional judgement in relation to the level of risk Alice was facing.

Harry Douglass (2005), writing about practice theory for adult protection, develops the helpful concept of 'sensitive authority' as a middle way between an overly managerial, mechanistic approach and a dismissive or trivialising response to safeguarding. This 'middle way' is not an easy choice, entailing as it does engagement with uncertainty and the inevitability of risk taking. As Douglass (p. 42) argues:

> Intervention that combines empathy, sensitivity and a desire to empower individuals in crisis with sound professional judgement and informed decision making within a transparent procedural framework is most likely to afford the necessary protection to an adult vulnerable to abuse.

Sue was consistently clear that changes needed to take place if Alice was to remain at home with her family. In this situation confident 'sensitive authority', combined with a clear sense of her professional and statutory role, enabled Sue to negotiate an outcome where risk was acknowledged and managed in a way that respected the individual biographies and the family system of those involved.

Sue's intervention was never likely to be about 'solving' a problem. Alice's deteriorating health meant that the solutions she was able to negotiate with Michael, Ellen and other family members were inevitably short term. Her involvement was however crucial in transforming a situation of high risk to one of acceptable risk, The close attention to the rights and choices of those involved, which was central to Sue's approach, also meant that Alice's final, inevitable move to a nursing home happened in a context of acceptance and agreement rather than conflict and failure.

12 Fiona, Jack and Esther: Supporting Unwise Decisions

Questions to ask yourself as you read:

- Why is it sometimes important to support people's unwise decisions?

- What are some of the challenges of working with older people who support disabled adult children?

- Do you think that any more could have been done to promote Esther or Jack's best interests?

Fiona, Jack and Esther

Fiona, an experienced social worker in a community team, received a referral from a local general practitioner (GP) concerned about Esther, a 76-year-old woman who lived with her 40-year-old son Jack. According to the GP, Jack had a mild learning disability, which was 'probably Aspergers'. Although he had been to a special school, there was no record of Jack having received social care services as an adult. Esther had recently sent the GP a letter which said that following the recent death of her husband, she was struggling with her own deteriorating mobility and with having to look after Jack. The GP was particularly concerned as Esther had recently been diagnosed with breast cancer and was reluctant to accept treatment.

Fiona made several phone calls to Esther over the next few weeks, but Esther consistently refused either to allow Fiona to visit or to agree to a meeting elsewhere. She said that the letter to the GP was a 'mistake' and she and Jack were 'muddling through'. Fiona admits that according to formal agency procedures, she should probably have closed the case at that point. However, a sense that all was not well with Esther and Jack meant that she continued trying to make contact:

> I phoned four or five times before Esther eventually agreed to a visit. I got the feeling that she was quite glad to talk to someone and although she said she didn't want help, I somehow wasn't convinced that she meant it. I also felt she was very fearful and anxious and I wasn't sure why.

Fiona attempted to visit Esther at the agreed time, but there was no response to her knock on the door. Fiona noticed that there were several broken, boarded up windows in the house. A neighbour told her that the damage had been done by Jack who had 'lost it' one day. According to the neighbour, Jack was prone to outbursts of shouting and this was not the first time he had done damage to the house. Although the neighbour had offered to call the police, Esther had been very clear that she had not been harmed and did not want the police involved.

Fiona was concerned enough by what she had seen and heard to return at a different time the following day:

> I took them by surprise when I called, but it seemed the only way I was going to get to see them. It took me a while to negotiate my way into the house. I had to tread very, very carefully. Esther was extremely anxious and fearful and didn't want me to talk to Jack. Jack was quite hostile and upset that my visit had disturbed his daily routine. Once I was inside the house, there was no disguising the fact that Jack was prone to angry and violent outbursts — there were holes in most of the doors and the kitchen cupboards where he'd kicked them. It was a pretty unsafe environment.

The state of the house and the evidence of Jack's extreme temper were such that Fiona felt Esther was potentially at risk of harm. After discussions between Fiona and her manager and with Jack and Esther's GP, it was decided that the case should be considered under the local authority's procedure for the safeguarding of vulnerable adults:

> It was complicated because they were actually both very vulnerable. In the end there wasn't any evidence of physical abuse towards Esther, but Jack's outbursts were physically dangerous and emotionally upsetting to her. So there was a safeguarding investigation and a protection plan was put in place.

In fact, Jack surprised everyone by being unexpectedly willing to accept services himself as part of the protection plan put in place to safeguard his mother. Fiona managed to introduce a social worker and a psychologist from the learning disability team who gradually began to find ways to support Jack and to help him find new activities outside the home. Fiona also got help from a local voluntary organisation to undertake repairs and redecorate Esther and Jack's house.

Esther and Jack's situation was much improved. Jack was becoming calmer and more socially integrated, the house was in a better state of repair and various small adaptations had enabled Esther to move around her home more easily and safely. In spite of this, as she got to know Esther and Jack better, Fiona became increasingly aware of the complexity of the family dynamics and the ongoing difficulties that that they were facing.

> They had both been floundering after Jack's dad died. He had clearly been the dominant member of the household and I'm pretty sure he had been violent towards both of them. There was another son who had left home at a young age and refused to have anything to do with the family since; that made me even more concerned about what had gone on in the past...
>
> ... Once we'd got to know each other, Jack was more open about his mood swings than Esther and actually more willing to accept help than she was. She was very frightened of letting Jack out of her sight and insisted he wouldn't cope with the social and educational activities he was being encouraged to take part in.

Although Jack was approaching middle age, he had never really had an independent life or friends of his own and his movements outside the home had been strictly controlled by his father. For Jack to be spending time away from his mother, doing things he had chosen to do himself was a massive life change not only for him, but also for Esther. Unfortunately, while Jack seemed to be thriving on the new opportunities that were opening up to him, Esther was struggling.

> I was working quite closely with the learning disability social worker who was now working with Jack. He was doing this really satisfying piece of work and Jack was getting involved in all sorts of new things. Meanwhile I was getting nowhere with Esther. She seemed more anxious about Jack every day and she was still refusing to go into hospital for breast cancer treatment. I assessed her

capacity more than once, but it was very clear that she was able to make up her own mind about this. I had to respect her decision and go with it, so did the GP and the district nurse, who was also involved by this point. We all tried to help her see the benefits of getting treatment and found ways of trying to alleviate her anxiety about Jack, but she'd sort of stopped listening and put up a barrier that we couldn't break through. I stayed involved because of the safeguarding plan that was in place, but there wasn't much I could do. It was a bit of a waiting game.

Fiona clearly felt frustrated by what she felt to be a lack of progress in her work with Esther. Jack seemed to be embracing change and thriving on it, while Esther was becoming both more anxious and more determined to accept as little outside intervention as possible. Eventually, Esther's deteriorating health led inevitably to a change in her situation. Esther collapsed at home and was admitted to hospital, where she was treated for minor injuries associated with her fall. Once in hospital Esther agreed to surgery and chemotherapy for her breast cancer. Fiona became involved once more when, after a period of rehabilitation Esther was ready to be discharged from hospital:

Being in hospital was obviously a good thing for Esther's physical health, but it seemed to do her mental health some good too. She was less caught up in her day to day anxieties about what Jack was doing and actually Jack was doing ok. There were a few setbacks along the way, but the social worker working with him set up quite a bit of support while his mum was in hospital and anyway Jack was becoming more independent than any of us had really thought possible.

Fiona worked with Esther for several weeks while she was still in hospital and then made arrangements for her to go to a residential home for a short period of further rehabilitation. Fiona was able to argue for this resource on the basis of the earlier safeguarding concerns and the fact that in her current physically fragile state, Esther would be particularly vulnerable to any physically aggressive outbursts from Jack.

She thrived in the home. Having a structure and routine seemed to suit her. She made friends and developed some really good relationships with the staff. Her care needs were quite considerable though and that didn't really change. Her general frailty and limited mobility meant that she would have been eligible to stay there permanently and for a while she had pretty much decided to do that. I thought it was the perfect solution. A good outcome for everyone.

Fiona spent time helping Esther to plan a permanent move to the residential home. She liaised with Jack's social worker and with Jack himself to reassure Esther that her son would be safe and supported without her as well as helping to sort out the necessary legal and financial arrangements. However, just days before the move was due to become permanent, Esther changed her mind and decided that she wanted to go home after all. Fiona admits that she was deeply disappointed with this outcome.

> I'd seen a dramatic change for the better in Esther while she'd been in the home and the reports on Jack were great – way beyond anyone's expectations. Then suddenly what had seemed like a really good piece of work was coming apart at the seams. Esther was full of anxiety again and I had to do the best I could to put together a package of care that she would agree to that would meet her needs and dovetail with the support that Jack was receiving.

Esther returned home a couple of weeks later with quite a complex package of support. In order to arrange this Fiona had to negotiate carefully with Esther herself and with several health colleagues who were increasingly involved in Esther's care. In addition she had to work closely with the social worker and others who were supporting Jack, in order not to jeopardise the progress he had made towards increasing independence. For Fiona, the sense that this was perhaps not the best outcome for either Esther or Jack remained. However, Fiona also recognised Esther's right to make decisions about her own life and the importance of not imposing solutions, however strongly she might have felt that it would have been in Esther's best interests to do so.

> I stayed involved with Esther and Jack until she died about 9 months later. It was a house full of stress, conflict and anxiety until the end. Everyone involved tried to make it as calm and as safe as it could be for Esther – that was all we could do. Maybe I should have tried harder to persuade her to stay in the care home, but in the end she was an adult with the capacity to make her own decisions and I had to respect that.

Discussion

In her work with Jack and Esther, Fiona was involved in a situation characterised by conflict, anxiety and feelings of ambivalence. Inevitably, this impacted on both the process and the outcome of her practice. Unlike some of the social work stories in this book, the intervention described here did not result in a straightforwardly positive conclusion. Social work practice inevitably reflects the ambiguities of real life and what is best in practice is revealed not so much in the outcome as in the way the social worker manages the resulting complexity.

As we discussed in Chapter 1, even the most thoughtful, self-aware and well informed practice does not lead inevitably to a result that everyone involved would define as 'good'. Fiona's disappointment with the final outcome of her work was evident from the way she spoke about it. Nevertheless much of the process of her intervention with Esther and Jack was

> the best that was achieved at that time, in that situation, by that combination of people, processes and circumstances. (Jones et al., 2008a, p. 4)

Recognising the unpredictable nature of social work practice is essential to an understanding of the complexity of the social work task. The fact that the final result of an intervention does not necessarily reflect the quality of the practice that has taken place means that social work can never be measured or calculated solely in terms of outcomes. As Barry Cooper argues:

> 'Best' practices cannot be defined by a judgement of outcome. Social realities and the nature of social work interventions are too complex and the identification of 'outcomes' too open ended and ambiguous for this to be a fair or representative measure of social work. (Cooper, 2008, p. 122)

Once Esther was settled and apparently contented in the residential home and Jack was developing his own independence so successfully, Fiona hoped and believed that she had secured an effective outcome to her intervention. Nevertheless Esther decided to return home. While this was not the option that Fiona would have chosen or the one that she believed to be in Esther's best interests, she recognised Esther's right and capacity to make her own informed decision and supported her choice. Under the circumstances this was probably the best practice that could be achieved at the time, in that particular situation even though the outcome involved Esther's return to a stressful and often difficult home environment.

Terry O'Sullivan (2011, p. 11), writing about decision making in social work, distinguishes between 'sound' decisions, which relate to the process of practice, and 'effective' decisions, which relate to outcomes. While the first will in many cases lead to the second, the uncertainty involved in any decision-making process means that outcomes are never wholly predictable. O'Sullivan's recipe for sound decision making comprises critical awareness of context, user involvement, collaboration, using knowledge and managing emotions, framing decisions in a clear, accurate way, analysing options and using supervision effectively. While this may feel like a long list and a lot to ask of an individual practitioner, it not only summarises rather accurately Fiona's work in this situation, but also that of most of the other social workers whose practice is presented in this book.

All the older people in this section were also parents of adult children with whom they had complex relationships. Esther, like Alice in the previous chapter, was an older woman with her own social, emotional and health needs. However, her sense of herself, her role and her responsibilities was also deeply entwined in her relationship with her son Jack. A post-structural perspective, which resists the idea of fixed identity and recognises that people can see themselves as several things at once, is a helpful way for practitioners to understand and work with the seeming ambiguity of 'multiple and often contradictory identifications' (Healy, 2005, p. 210). Esther's feelings towards her son were complex and ambiguous. Sometimes she saw Jack as a threat and was acutely aware of her own vulnerability and ill health. At other times Esther seemed to feel either that she needed to supervise and control Jack's behaviour or that she needed to protect him from the outside world. This sometimes contradictory reaction was further complicated by the dramatic shift in Jack's own identity, behaviour and attitude as he became increasingly independent.

Part of the strength of Fiona's practice was her ability to recognise and work with changing dynamics and competing needs. The internal conflict that Esther was experiencing engendered some apparently contradictory decisions and changes of mind on her part. We know less about Jack as Fiona spent only a short time working with him directly. However, some of the good outcomes for Jack, such as his increasing independence, were seemingly difficult and stressful for Esther, while her insistence on remaining at home limited Jack's ability to control his own life. Social work decisions sometimes inevitably involve outcomes that may be good for one person and far less satisfactory for another what O'Sullivan (2011, p. 177) calls 'competing claims within decision situations'. It is hardly surprising then that Adams et al. (2009, p. 6) talk about social work as the 'complexity profession' and emphasise 'complexity thinking' as the most appropriate course of action for a social worker to take. They define this as

> inclusive thinking, holding within it the logic that enables us to hold competing claims and contradictions while looking for solutions. We look for alternatives and different sides of the situation and integrate them into a discourse. (p. 7)

Fiona could have walked away from this case without ever meeting Esther or Jack if she had interpreted Esther's initial refusal to see her simply as a matter of choice and straightforward rejection of the service being offered. Instead, Fiona's recognition that the situation was more complicated than it seemed led to a quiet persistence in finding ways to establish a relationship with Esther and Jack. Similarly Fiona's growing understanding of the relationship between mother and son ensured that although she made appropriate use of local authority safeguarding procedures to protect Esther, she simultaneously recognised Jack's vulnerability and need for support. Fiona therefore rejected the sort of 'binary oppositional thinking' (Jones and Powell, 2008, p. 64), which can lead to the simplification or surface interpretation of events, in favour of the sort of 'inclusive' 'complexity thinking' that Adams et al. advocate.

As she came to know Esther and Jack better, Fiona's suspicion that Esther's husband had been exceptionally domineering and controlling of both of them became stronger. Neither Esther nor Jack appeared to have any experience of making decisions for themselves or for each other. However, while Jack embraced his newly acquired independence and choice, Esther fluctuated between welcoming and rejecting change, often expressing guilt for failing to keep things as they had always been. In spite of invitations to do so, Esther would tell Fiona very little about her past life. Nevertheless Fiona became close enough to both Jack and Esther to understand that they had undergone difficult and damaging past experiences and to recognise the care and caution needed in order to establish a working relationship.

Jack and Esther's situation was particularly complex and challenging. However, the frequency with which difficulties arise in planning for the future where adults with learning difficulties live at home with elderly parents has been well documented. In their research study Bowey and McGlaughin (2007) found that about half of the older carers of adults with learning difficulties that they talked to were either unready or unwilling to make future plans. Other writers and researchers have highlighted the 'system of mutual dependence' (Lindsay, 2008) that often arises in such situations and the failure of policy makers to recognise the significance of these reciprocal caring relationships (Parker and Clarke, 2002). Esther's life had been deeply entwined with Jack's for more than 40 years. Although there was much about their shared past that remained unknown to Fiona, it was essential for her to consider their needs individually and together in order to work with what Bowey and McGlaughin (2005, p. 1379) term 'the mutuality of the relationship'.

There were hints from both Esther and Jack that their family life had been overshadowed by violence and the controlling behaviour of Jack's father. Fiona tried to open up conversations about the past with Esther, but with little success:

> Esther would say that the past was 'best left where it was'. I knew enough to be sure I had to tread carefully and sensitively, but there was clearly a lot of pain and fear associated with things in her marriage that I didn't know about. In an ideal world we might have found the space to be able to explore the past in more depth, but the priority had to be to keep them both safe and give them support and some choices for the future.

Fiona worked hard to build a relationship with Esther and Jack that was sufficiently trusting for her to be able to negotiate changes and introduce a range of health and social care services. This was essentially a forward-looking, problem-solving approach rather than one which sought to explore Esther and Jack's past experiences. Anne Weick (1989, p. 251), writing about strengths-based approaches, asserts the value of this when she argues that 'Concern about establishing the precise cause of the problem ensnares social workers in a strategy for dealing with the problem in those terms'. As Fiona reflected on her work with Esther, she continued to wonder whether spending more time 'establishing the precise cause of the problem' would in fact have led to Esther making different choices in the present and an outcome that might have been judged more effective. However, part of what Fiona did so well in this situation was to support Esther to accept the help and make the changes she was ready for, in her own time and on her own terms. Esther had the capacity to make her own decisions and as section 1 of the Mental Capacity Act 2005 makes clear: 'A person is not to be treated as unable to make a decision merely because he makes an unwise decision'.

While Fiona continued to feel that it would have been in Esther's best interests to remain in the residential home, there can be little doubt that her intervention made a real and positive difference to the lives of both Esther and Jack. Fiona's intervention therefore resonates strongly with an interpretation of 'best practice' which

> [d]oes not mean 'this could have been best if only this, that or the other had been the case'. It is recognising the actualities of practice, within which 'best' is simply the best that could have been achieved at the time. It is 'best' taking a reality check. 'Best' in terms of what was achieved despite and because of all the complexities and difficulties. (Jones et al., 2008b, p. 288)

In spite of Fiona's reservations about the outcome of her involvement, she did the 'best' she could under the circumstances. This was a situation after all, within which the risk to Esther was managed and she was enabled to live with reasonable safety in a situation of her own choosing. For Jack there can be little doubt that the introduction of outside support leading to a degree of independence which would not otherwise have been possible represented real and positive change.

13 Judy and Dorothy: The Older Person as Expert

Questions to ask yourself as you read:

- In what ways was this intervention shaped by Dorothy's strengths?
- How far should family members be expected to provide care?
- Why is a 'critical' approach important in social work practice?

Judy and Dorothy

Dorothy had been assessed by several different members of the older adults community team, over a period of some years, when she was referred to Judy, a senior social worker:

> I knew of Dorothy, but I'd never met her. Various social workers and occupational therapists had been involved at different points and I'd heard a lot of stories about her, so although I tried to go in with an open mind, I had an idea of her as someone who was quite eccentric.

Dorothy was in her mid-nineties when she and Judy first met. She had a diagnosis of schizophrenia which dated back to the 1960s, but she wasn't taking any medication or receiving specific treatment for this condition. Dorothy was getting daily help with shopping and some aspects of personal care funded by the local authority. It was the care agency providing this support that made a referral to Judy's team, reporting that Dorothy's behaviour had become increasingly bizarre.

According to the carers, Dorothy's strange behaviour included urinating in a bowl or on newspaper rather than in the toilet, drying incontinence pads under the grill, eating and drinking erratically and refusing to eat food prepared by the carers. They were also concerned that Dorothy was boiling water in a saucepan, rather than using the kettle and they feared that she might scald herself.

Judy recognised the sensitivity of some of these issues and was determined to approach her first meeting with Dorothy with caution:

> *I was prepared for this really difficult conversation, but actually it wasn't too bad. I'm not sure that anyone had ever asked Dorothy in detail what her life was like and she was surprisingly keen to talk about. She had been carrying around this 'mad old lady' label for decades and I think it really got in the way of people being able to take what she said seriously. I mean, yes she had some strange mannerisms and she'd sometimes talk very quickly or go off at odd tangents, but when you got through that she could give a pretty clear account of her day-to-day life, how she coped and what she needed.*

As Judy worked with Dorothy to unpick the issues outlined in the referral from the care agency, she came to see a pattern emerging:

> *There was an explanation for everything – a kind of logic and rationality at the heart of all she did. I challenged some of the outcomes of that logic because I felt she was putting herself at risk, but actually she didn't do anything without a good reason. Yet the perception of those around her was quite the opposite – that nothing she did made any sense. She had no intention of changing most of her behaviour though. In fact I think she sometimes exaggerated it just to annoy people.*

During her initial assessment, Judy established that Dorothy's arthritis meant that she found it physically more comfortable to urinate into a bowl and then tip the contents down the toilet. She would also pad herself with newspaper 'just in case' the incontinence pad proved inadequate. Because of the lack of strength in her arms and fingers, she found it easier to slide a saucepan off the stove than to lift an electric kettle. The reason for drying her incontinence pads under the grill was because, according to Dorothy, 'someone' had told her she was not allowed to put anything wet into the bin. Finally, although her eating routine was certainly unusual and included some food combinations that most people would find strange, she was actually very much in control of her own needs and routines:

> *In some ways she was the epitome of the 'expert patient'. She knew what she needed to eat and when, in order to manage her recurring constipation without medication. She had arthritis, but she knew how she needed to manage things around the house in order to be able to cope with very little outside help.*

As Judy began to establish a relationship of trust with Dorothy, she was able to correct some of her long-held misconceptions and to make suggestions and recommendations, some of which were accepted, while others were refused.

> After a while, when I got to know Dorothy better, she took it from me that it was ok to wrap up wet incontinence pads and put them in the bin. She still used newspaper as well, insisting it was a 'tried and tested method', but I did at least get her to put this in a plastic bag before she threw it away. I got an occupational therapist involved and she organised a toilet frame, which was a great help. She also got Dorothy a new kettle which was much safer and easier to use, but Dorothy still preferred the saucepan. In the end I had to make a judgement – about her capacity to make her own decisions and about her safety. There were more things I'd like to have changed at this point, but I didn't feel she was unsafe and I actually thought she was much more able to make her own decisions than people had given her credit for.

Judy doubted that Dorothy's diagnosis of schizophrenia had ever been accurate, but in spite of more than one past psychiatric referral, no one had ever seemed able to provide a more helpful diagnosis. Judy did not feel that this was likely to be a productive route to go down again:

> She was clearly familiar with (and very dismissive of) psychiatric services. She adamantly rejected the idea of a psychiatric referral and I felt that not much would be gained by it. The main thing was to keep her safe and give her some choice and control over her life.

Dorothy had a daughter, Mae, who was in her sixties and lived locally. Mae had her own health problems, but she visited her mother weekly and took care of her finances and other paperwork. Judy spent time with Mae, who told her quite a lot about Dorothy's past life:

> Mae told me her mum had always been 'difficult'. She said that when she was younger, Dorothy would sometimes fly into furious rages with very little provocation. She talked about how Mae and her sister had been left on their own while Dorothy disappeared to London for weeks. According to Mae there had been several different men around during her childhood, but neither she nor her sister were sure who their father was and Dorothy still refused to say. Yet Dorothy had also held some responsible jobs, working as a secretary in the war office in the 1940s and later in a number of administrative roles, but periodically there would be some sort of 'incident' and another job would be lost...

...I wondered whether Mae would agree to be more involved in her mother's care as she got older and frailer, but there was just no way. Their relationship was full of conflict and quite a lot of pain. I tried to get them to talk to each other, but I was working against decades of conflict and neither of them seemed to want to change things.

Judy worked with Dorothy to make changes to her package of care. As well as the occupational therapy assessment, she negotiated some small changes to the timing and nature of the care Dorothy was receiving and talked to the care workers about their concerns and how these had been addressed.

For over a year, the situation seemed stable, but then Dorothy, by now aged nearly 97, slipped on the ice in her garden and fell and broke her leg:

Poor Dorothy wasn't in a good state when I first visited her in hospital. She had got very cold lying on the ground waiting for the ambulance to arrive and she was badly bruised and still in quite a lot of pain. I don't think any of us – not me, not the ward staff, the doctors or Dorothy's daughter thought she would ever be able to go home.

Dorothy spent several weeks in hospital and then moved to a nursing home where she underwent a programme of rehabilitation. Almost nine months after her fall, she was now able to stand and walk a few steps, but with greatly reduced mobility, Dorothy insisted that she was ready to return home. Once again her capacity to make this decision became an issue:

The district nurse wanted nothing to do with the idea of Dorothy living independently again. She felt strongly that she wasn't able to make that decision. The manager of the nursing home was very supportive though – I don't think that was only because Dorothy was far from the easiest resident she'd ever had! I assessed her capacity again and on this particular decision about living independently, I felt she was well able to make an informed choice.

Judy co-ordinated a full multi-professional assessment, with staff from the nursing home, the occupational therapist and the physiotherapist involved in Dorothy's rehabilitation, Dorothy's general practitioner (GP) and albeit reluctantly, her district nurse. Dorothy's daughter Mae was also involved in the assessment. Mae was clear that she was not in a position to provide any more care for her mother than she had in the past. However, although she would have preferred Dorothy to remain

139

in the nursing home, she was broadly supportive of her mother's right to make her own decisions.

As the assessment progressed, it became clear that given her increased mobility problems, Dorothy's current flat was no longer going to be suitable for her. At this point, a housing officer became closely involved and working together with Dorothy; he and Judy were able to identify a bungalow in an 'extra care' housing scheme, which they felt would meet Dorothy's needs:

> It was fortunate that the bungalow became available when it did. It was fully adapted and there were care staff on site to pop in and help Dorothy two or three times a day. And... most important of all, she loved it.

So Dorothy moved in to her new bungalow with an intensive package of support. By this point Judy had known Dorothy on and off for several years. This inevitably helped her to prepare the ground with the manager of the housing scheme and the care staff who were to be working with Dorothy:

> I was able to talk to the manager about some of the issues that had arisen in the past and tell her a bit about what to expect when she met Dorothy. I don't know whether that helped or whether it was more to do with the fact that Dorothy was so pleased about the move, but they formed a pretty good relationship.

At the time of writing, Dorothy who is now 101 has been living in her 'extra care' bungalow for three years. Judy has been involved intermittently during that period:

> There have been difficulties of course. Sometimes I've been involved in mediation between Dorothy and Mae. Like the time Dorothy fell out with care staff, packed her bags and turned up at Mae's one-bedroom flat. She couldn't get into it of course because it was up a flight of stairs and I'm not sure Mae would have let her in anyway. Another time, Dorothy decided she was being poisoned by the central heating and refused to turn it on. It was freezing and she ended up wearing just about every item of clothing she had. The manager was sure Dorothy was going to die of hypothermia. In fact, when we managed to get her talk about it, it turned out that she had a friend who died of carbon monoxide poisoning so as usual there was a logical explanation for her behaviour, even if it was filtered through Dorothy's particular way of seeing the world. When we explained that she could get a carbon monoxide monitor, she accepted it and turned the heating back on.

Discussion

It would be difficult to argue that the practice which took place here was dominated by 'difference and disagreement', the topic of this section of the book. Judy's work with Dorothy was empathetic, open, person-centred and effective. However, it is included here because on this occasion, skilled practice helped prevent the conflict that had dominated earlier professional interventions in Dorothy's life and could so easily have arisen again.

Judy herself was expecting to encounter someone who was 'difficult' and 'eccentric', indeed her position as a senior practitioner meant that most of the cases allocated to her were by definition challenging or problematic. In spite of this, Judy met Dorothy with an open mind. She was prepared to make her own assessment of Dorothy's behaviour and of her mental health and to plan her intervention accordingly. In this respect, Judy's practice exemplified the sort of open, questioning and thoughtful practice associated with a critical approach to social work. Malcolm Payne (2012, p. 108), writing about what he calls 'citizenship social work' with older people, frames his analysis of critical thinking in terms of the following:

- *Critical analysis of language.* This involves thinking about the most appropriate ways of communicating and leaving space for the older person's narrative or story.

- *Avoiding taken-for-granted assumptions in practice.* In other words, questioning accepted categories, definitions and ways of doing things.

- *Critical discourse analysis.* That is, the deconstruction of discussion and disagreement between people to get beneath the surface of talk and understand the power relations between people.

Judy's practice exemplified all three elements of Payne's definition. From their first meeting, Judy took an open-minded, reflexive approach to her conversations with Dorothy, which allowed her space to tell the story of her day-to-day life in her own way. Such an approach contrasts with the uncritical application of agency questionnaires and procedures that sometimes characterises practice with older people. As Anne Weick et al. (1989, p. 351) point out, this sort of agency led proceduralism encourages the 'matching' of clients to predetermined categories and can mean that the idiosyncratic characteristics, which say most about a person, are overlooked. In the situation described in this chapter, Judy's open mindedness involved taking the reports of Dorothy's behaviour as serious cause for concern, but also recognising that the representation of Dorothy's actions as 'strange and bizarre' was just one way of understanding what was going on. By engaging with Dorothy's own narrative, Judy understood that behaviour, which might have been categorised as 'mad' or 'dangerous', could equally be interpreted as rational and carefully planned.

Nigel Parton (2003, p. 9) defines the sort of critical reflexivity, which avoids 'taken for granted assumptions' as

> the continual attempt to place one's premises into question and to listen to alternative framings of reality in order to grapple with the potentially different outcomes arising out of different points of view.

Judy was aware of Dorothy's 'eccentric' reputation, her long-standing, but questionable diagnosis of schizophrenia and the fact that several fellow professionals had struggled to work effectively with her. This was important information which helped Judy prepare for her first meeting with Dorothy, but which nevertheless remained open to question. Judy resisted taking others' interpretations of Dorothy's behaviour for granted, using them instead as contributions in the process of establishing her own assessment of Dorothy's situation. Through her ability to 'reflect heretically' (Adams et al., 2009, p. 4) in this way, Judy came to understand that Dorothy's supposed eccentricity was part of a need to control her own life and her own situation. Much of Dorothy's behaviour, including her frequent disputes with health and social care professionals, arose from a refusal to acquiesce to taken-for-granted assumptions about how a very elderly, physically frail woman should behave.

Judy spoke about her work with Dorothy with warmth, enthusiasm and occasionally with exasperation. During the several years they have known each other, Judy has been called upon to mediate in many disputes involving Dorothy and members of her family, neighbours or health and welfare professionals. These situations have not always reflected well on Dorothy; indeed Judy is clear that Dorothy is someone who has demanded more time, patience and tolerance than almost any of her other clients. In spite of this, Judy has engaged imaginatively with Dorothy's situation, seeking to understand her perspective and use her many strengths to improve Dorothy's quality of life on her own terms.

Denis Saleeby's definition of the 'strengths based' practitioner resonates strongly with Judy's approach:

> the social work practitioner must be genuinely interested in, and respectful of clients' stories, narratives and accounts – the interpretive angles they take on their own experiences. (Saleeby, 2006, p. 16)

By attending carefully and with authentic interest and concern to Dorothy's own explanation of her lifestyle, Judy was able to see beyond the negative labels and assumptions that had been attached to Dorothy. This did not mean that there were no issues, tensions or areas of disagreement between them. It did mean, however, that Judy was able to move beyond a deficit approach and to work collaboratively with Dorothy to ensure that her future was planned on her own terms.

Strengths-based approaches are often described as moving away from 'pathologising' the client or service user (Healy, 2005, p. 154) to a more optimistic way of working, which both reflects and build on the service user's capacity. This sort of future-orientated practice is often not used in a considered way with older people, who are by definition moving towards the end of their lives. However Dorothy, like many older people, was an expert in her own experience and had strong views on the best way of managing her own health and daily living needs. The conflict and disagreement, which characterised her interactions with health and social care practitioners, tended to result from attempts to impose a solution or interpretation that differed from Dorothy's own. This meant that Judy's role was often that of 'mediator translator' (Weick et al. 1989, p. 354) or 'translator' (Payne, 2012, p. 52) helping to build solutions which placed Dorothy's strengths and self-knowledge at the centre of decisions about her welfare.

Through her critical approach, Judy was able to take on board earlier assessments and reports of Dorothy's needs, while continually questioning and scrutinising them. Dorothy's 50-year-old diagnosis of schizophrenia seemed to be largely without foundation, yet it had provided a powerful lens through which several of those involved in her care had viewed Dorothy's behaviour. Additionally, Dorothy's advanced age brought with it expectations about dependency and passivity which had coloured the thinking of most people encountering the physically frail 90-year-old. Most of us are susceptible to these sorts of assumptions and stereotypes but as Judy recognised, Dorothy's rejection of them was central to her sense of herself. Karen Healy (2005, p. 208) proposes a narrative approach as a way of separating the person from the problem so that the problem or the need does not become the only way in which someone is identified:

> Narrative therapy aims to reconstruct the dominant narratives that shape the service user's life from those that emphasize pathology to those that highlight and support the service user's capacities.

Judy's ability to support Dorothy's capacities and to act as an advocate or a translator in the process of planning her future was central in reducing the conflict and disagreement that had so often surrounded the care services she received.

Dorothy's independence and determination to define her own needs were at the heart of the way in which Judy engaged with her. At the same time however, Dorothy's frailty and the possibility that she might come to physical harm was an ongoing concern to Judy and a cause of disagreement between the professionals involved in Dorothy's care. This tension between protection and the right of the individual to choose to take risks is almost always present in social work with older people and does not lend itself to easy or simplistic solutions. Judy undertook several assessments of Dorothy's capacity to make specific decisions, as she was required to do under the Mental Capacity Act 2005 and assured herself as fully as she could that Dorothy was able to make these decisions. However, Judy was also aware that even the best mental capacity assessment is not an infallible process and can result in a 'simplistic dichotomy between people being deemed to have or lack capacity' (Mantell and Clark, 2011, p. 60). She was therefore committed to working with Dorothy in order to minimise the dangers she was facing and to negotiate ways of reducing risk. By establishing a relationship of confidence and trust, many of Judy's suggestions that there were safer ways in which Dorothy might manage some activities of daily life were accepted. These deceptively straightforward outcomes contrasted with Dorothy's previous conflictual relationships with health and social care professionals, most of which had resulted in her refusal to consider any change or compromise.

Part of Judy's skill was her ability to work creatively with the notion of risk taking, rather than viewing it simply as something to be eliminated. It has sometimes been argued that the concept of risk in social work has become overly associated with danger and this has, in turn, led to defensive and risk-avoidant practice (Thompson, 2000; Parton,

2003; Cree and Wallace, 2009). An approach that is characterised by the notion of 'better safe than sorry' (Smethurst, 2011, p. 174) may be well meaning, but the consequences can be oppressive for the service user and likely to compromise autonomy and self determination. Dorothy would probably have been less physically at risk if Judy had used the relationship they had established to convince Dorothy to move permanently to a nursing home. Judy herself admitted that this outcome would have given her 'fewer sleepless nights'; however, it would also have compromised the independence that meant more to Dorothy than anything else.

The idea of 'positive risk taking' (Gaylard, 2009) offers a way of reframing the conventional view of risk as a threat or danger and ensuring that the focus of social work intervention is not just about minimising risk, but about maximising welfare (Munro, 2002). Judy supported Dorothy's independence and insistence on doing things in her own way, because she recognised that these were important aspects of her identity and therefore central to her well-being. This was a critical approach to risk analysis, which involved weighing up the potential benefits and harms of exercising one choice or action over another. By valuing Dorothy's life choices, Judy resisted simplistic calculations of risk, which might have led to Dorothy being physically safer, but would probably also have had a negative impact on her welfare.

An approach like Judy's acknowledges the unpredictability and uncertainty of life and recognises that social work intervention can never provide a 'quick fix' solution (Cree and Wallace, 2009, p. 42). As several writers have argued, it does sometimes feel as though social work policy makers and managers have generated increasingly restrictive procedures, including risk management tools in an attempt to reduce or eliminate complexity and uncertainty (McBeath and Webb, 2002; Webb, 2006). Wilson et al. (2011, p. 7) point out that while these sorts of managerial approaches have their place, they are 'incomplete responses to the conditions they are seeking to address'. Judy did not minimise the issue of risk in her work with Dorothy, but she did recognise the potential of risk taking in terms of Dorothy's treasured independence and autonomy. This involved embracing unpredictability and uncertainty as part of a positive choice on Dorothy's part rather than simplistically seeking to eliminate it.

The tension between self-determination and the responsibility to protect was a cause of difference and disagreement between those involved in Dorothy's care and between Dorothy herself and the professionals she encountered. These tensions are themselves part of the uncertainty and unpredictability of social work. By practicing in an open and critical way however, Judy was able to resist taken-for-granted assumptions about how Dorothy ought to behave. She used a flexible, strengths-oriented approach, which recognised that in many situations the elimination of risk is neither possible nor desirable (O'Sullivan, 2011, p. 116). By allowing the possibility of risk taking as a positive and welfare-enhancing activity, Judy was able to work with Dorothy's own choices and preferences. The result of this was not only to reduce the amount of conflict in Dorothy's dealings with social care staff, but also to make her safer. The importance of positive risk taking is a recurring theme in the stories in this book and is explored further in the next chapter, which considers issues of rights, risk and good judgement in social work practice.

Part 4

Rights, Risks and Good Judgement

14 Rights, Risks and Good Judgement

Introduction

It would be quite possible to analyse all the social work practice we have described in this book in terms of rights, risks and social workers' good judgement. In Chapter 8, we saw how Trish tried to ensure that Stella was not exploited financially whilst giving her as much control over her money as possible; Chapter 3 described Rachel's work with Michael, in which she slowly and carefully worked with him to introduce support on his own terms, allowing him to make the decisions. Maya, in Chapter 7, had to negotiate with Bill about accepting some support so that he could achieve his main aim of getting home as quickly as possible. The imperative to promote a client's rights and autonomy and yet to try to ensure that they do not come to harm is at the heart of what social workers do. It is built into our professional standards and ethics (The College of Social Work 2013; Health & Care Professionals Council, 2012) and woven into the fabric of day-to-day practice.

There are inevitably conflicts within a role which is required both to protect and to empower, so it is not surprising that the dilemmas that arise often cause social workers considerable difficulty. Humanistic approaches in social work stress the need to get alongside the people we work with and offer therapeutic, non-judgemental assistance. The emphasis is on understanding the other person's point of view and enabling them to come to their own conclusions rather than imposing our own – an approach which does not sit comfortably with duties to intervene in people's lives in order to protect them. Alongside the 'person-centred' traditions, social work is also deeply rooted in critical social theory. In radical or 'anti-oppressive' analysis, social workers find themselves in an uncomfortably paradoxical position, asserting the rights of the disadvantaged whilst wielding considerable power on behalf of a society in which that disadvantage is structurally entrenched.

Sometimes our powers are statutory, sometimes they are more nebulous, more a question of influence. But, how do you protect someone without limiting their autonomy? And when you do, whose interests are you serving? Is influence legitimate or is it always an abuse of power? Where does influence end and persuasion start? Social work has long recognised that there is 'a membrane so porous between caring and controlling that it dissolves at the slightest touch' (Sennett, 2003, p. 130).

In this chapter, we will pick up on some of the questions we started to explore in Chapter 2 about rights, vulnerability, authority and judgement, and discuss them further. We will then examine the issues at close quarters in the case studies that follow, showing how social workers negotiate the conflicts and paradoxes that arise in practice. In Chapter 15, Nada supports Joan to make a difficult decision about residential care and finds herself wrestling with the question of whether she has exerted too much influence over her client. We then move into more explicitly legal territory with Mr Wilson, who refuses much of the help he is offered and is assessed as lacking the capacity to decide how his care is provided. His social worker, Jane, works within the framework of Mental Capacity Act 2005 to come to a 'best interests' decision about his care. The last case study describes Matt's work with David, a man who has been 'kept safe' by his parents all his life but is encouraged by Matt to take risks and establish an independent life for himself.

The right to take risks

The rhetoric of individual rights and autonomy is now so central to mainstream social policy that it is easy to forget that this was not always the case. In their article 'Service Users and Practitioners Reunited', Beresford and Croft (2004) describe their unauthorised production in the 1980s of a report calling for the involvement of service users and community control of social services departments. Indeed, service user groups have fought for decades against state paternalism and interference, advocating a social model of disability and insisting that they themselves should be making decisions about their own lives. Much of this once controversial thinking has been absorbed into government policy, albeit within a much more market-driven and individualistic context than many of the service user movements anticipated.

Government policy initiatives are underpinned by an increasingly robust framework of legal rights. The Human Rights Act 1998, which came into force in 2000, made the edicts of the 1950 European Convention of Human Rights (ECHR) enforceable in British law courts. It gave people 'a clear legal statement of their basic rights and fundamental freedoms' (Great Britain, Department for Constitutional Affairs, 2006, p. 5) and placed a legal duty on public bodies to make the consideration of human rights part of all policy making and service delivery. Alongside this, the implementation of the Mental Capacity Act 2005 (MCA) has made the legal principles relating to individual decision-making very much clearer. There is a fundamental insistence that people who have the mental capacity to make decisions about their own lives have the legal right to do so, even if the decisions they make are unwise and put them in danger. Only when it is demonstrated that someone lacks the capacity to make a particular decision can a 'decision-maker' then decide, in consultation with others, what is in their best interests. Much of the MCA Code of Practice (Great Britain, Department for Constitutional Affairs, 2007) seeks to ensure that the decision-maker cannot act unilaterally, particularly when significant decisions are being made. They must consider the needs and wishes of the person themselves, consult with others, especially family, and under some circumstances an Independent Mental Capacity Advocate (IMCA) has to be appointed. Throughout the Mental Capacity Act, the emphasis is on limiting the powers of public bodies to intervene in people's lives in the name of 'protection'.

As we discussed in Chapter 2, current policies of 'personalisation' also stress the primacy of people's right to make decisions, if they have the capacity to do so, even when those decisions put them in danger. Safeguarding Adults procedures (Great Britain, Department of Health, 2000, 2009) make it clear that this applies even in situations where people are subject to abuse. There is a recognition that, with the pressures on social workers and other professionals to keep people safe, interventions can easily become over-protective. As we saw in the previous chapter, there are different ways of looking at the notion of 'risk'. On the one hand, you could argue that risks should be avoided so that there is less chance of harm or injury. On the other, and more positively, risks can been seen as actions that everyone has to take in order to progress and learn (Tulloch and Lupton, 2003). The argument is that social work has traditionally focused on the former at the expense of the latter and that there needs to be a conceptual shift away from 'risk avoidance' to 'risk enablement' and supporting people to take (sensible) risks (Great Britain, Department of Health, 2007b).

There clearly are ways in which 'protecting 'vulnerable' people from harm – although well intentioned – can be stifling' (Sayce, 2009, p. 104), and over-protectiveness can, paradoxically, increase the risks to someone's well-being. If in a bid for safety, people's lives become more constrained, their self-confidence may well diminish so that they feel more rather than less vulnerable. Keeping people safe can, all too easily, mean keeping them passive and socially excluded – they are more likely to be victims and less likely to speak out. However, if people are supported to take risks that enable them to do things that are important to them, this will increase their sense of autonomy and control and, ultimately, their safety (Sayce, 2009; Social Care Institute for Excellence, 2010). Our last case study in this section describes how Matt supports an older man called David, who is deaf and unable to speak. A little like Jack in Chapter 12, he had lived his whole life with his parents who 'kept him safe' by keeping him at home, almost completely cut off from the outside world. Matt works painstakingly with him to find a way of communicating and introducing him to life outside his home. In order to do this, he has to take risks – crossing roads, handling money, spending time on his own, meeting new people – and it is only by taking these risks that he starts to benefit from what life has to offer.

You can see a similar dynamic routinely at work in conventional approaches to service provision. Take the simple example of an older man who lives on his own and has always enjoyed going down to his local shops each day. He knows many of the shopkeepers and chats with them and other neighbours when he is out. After a stroke, he is no longer able to go out safely on his own, and the standard response is to arrange a shopping service to do it for him. He immediately loses a large part of his social life and his neighbours start to forget him, leaving him more isolated. He becomes depressed being stuck in the house all day and finds himself increasingly anxious, with nothing to distract him other than the television. He may be receiving his shopping safely but is, overall, considerably less safe and certainly less happy. A more positive approach to risk-taking would be to see how he could be supported to continue to go to the shops himself or, at least, to keep the vital links with his neighbourhood.

The reality of vulnerability

There is an obvious way in which this analysis of positive risk-taking is both true and central to good social work. And yet, there is also a sense in which a relentless emphasis on rights, choice and control fails to capture the extent of many people's vulnerability, especially when they are old and in poor health. The unprecedented value that Western culture gives to the ideal of individual autonomy has roots that stretch right back to the eighteenth-century Enlightenment. Being self-reliant, able to make our own decisions and govern our own lives in a rational and independent way has come almost to define what it means to be a citizen – even what it means to be a real person. Where adults seem unwilling to do this, they should be supported (or persuaded if they are unemployed and workshy) to be independent (Sennett, 2003). The difficulty is that, when independence is given so much value, those people who are dependent and vulnerable, and do need to be cared for, are rendered increasingly invisible. As Frost and Hoggett say,

> No role models, no icons, no social recognition exist for the very old. ... Old age in Western consumer societies is only defined as a deficit. (2008, p. 448)

Paradoxically, where positive, active images of ageing are used to counter ageist stereotypes, they may also appear to deny and devalue the very real physical, mental and emotional problems that exist for many people as they get old. In our personal lives, caring for the people close to us, feeling compassion, looking after those who are young or old or vulnerable is valued, and even considered essential. But the language of suffering and dependency seems to have slipped out of public policy. It is as if the discourse of individual rights and self-determination has effectively silenced the very human need for caring relationships, especially for those who, with age, become more physically and mentally frail.

These attitudes may stem from a collective denial of the reality that we all have physical limitations – that youth and health are not a given. Or it may be that our society is simply in thrall to its 'enchantment with cure' rather than the less dramatic 'women's work' of care (Hoggett, 2001, p. 44). But there is also a more hard-nosed, economic agenda. Dependency is expensive. Where people are paying for their own care, there seems to be no shame in choosing to move into a retirement village or care home or paying for a live-in carer or a companion. But, when the cost comes out of the public purse, the emphasis on rehabilitation and 'reablement' takes on distinctly moralising overtones, to the extent that not being independent (having 'no rehab. potential') is almost seen in terms of failure (Lloyd, 2006). Many older people will have internalised these values and so they themselves find the idea of being dependent ('a burden') somehow shameful. It is obvious, but significant, that the one decision that older people who need state funding are not allowed to make is that they would like to have more help and to be just a bit more dependent, to be cared for and looked after. The state typically only funds a care home place once someone is considered 'eligible' and it becomes the less expensive option. Live-in care, for older people who have no financial resources of their own, is very rare indeed.

So, whilst people have the right to take risks, the question is whether they are in a position in which they are able to make choices – even if, legally, they have the capacity to do so. It is easy to be seduced by the notion that people, ourselves included, make decisions by weighing up the pros and cons of a particular action and coming to a decision which takes all the factors into account. In this rational view of human nature, the role of the social worker would simply be to provide dispassionate, accurate information and ensure that someone understands the consequences of their decision. However, in reality, the decision-making process, especially at times of stress, is frequently too emotionally charged for this to be adequate. Psychologist Daniel Kahneman (2011) argues that, even at the best of times, human decision-making depends more on the knee-jerk reactions of (often flawed) intuitive feelings than it does on a considered and careful appraisal of the facts. And many older clients of social services, whilst having the capacity to make decisions, find their decision-making ability further impaired by their circumstances. As Liz Lloyd puts it:

> ... social workers' decisions about how best to assess and respond to need are taken at a time when an older person's capacity to engage in decision making is compromised by shattering events such as bereavement, moving house, serious illness and loss of mobility. (Lloyd, 2006, p. 1180)

If this is the case, then supporting a client to make a decision involves much more than presenting them with information and walking away.

Good judgement

Knowledge of law, policy, procedure and rights

By now, it should be clear that exercising good judgement in relation to rights and risks is always going to be a complex business for social workers. Cree and Wallace (2009, p. 45) have described a knowledge of law, policy and procedure and a commitment to rights as the four corners 'that should anchor good practice in relation to assessing and managing risk and protection'. As we have seen, it is often said that social work has become over-concerned with mechanised methods of assessment and risk management, that completing the correct forms within set timescales becomes more important than direct work with the client themselves. Practice can then become defensive as it focuses merely on demonstrating that the right procedures have been followed. There is certainly some truth in this and, especially as adult safeguarding moves on to a more legal footing, it seems unlikely to change. On the other hand, there is a difference between slavishly following procedure for procedure's sake and using law and policy clearly and explicitly to frame your work. Social work practice which is not clear about relevant law and policy, particularly in situations involving difficult judgements and risks, may not be defensive, but neither is it open to scrutiny and defensible. So, Safeguarding Adults guidance (Great Britain, Department of Health, 2000) is right to emphasise the importance of working with other professionals and good record keeping, ensuring that decision-making is shared, transparent and clearly documented. All of the social workers in the following section 'anchor' their work explicitly within the Mental Capacity Act 2005 and consider the rights of their clients and their own powers (or lack of powers) under this legislation. Jane uses powers under the Act to take Mr Wilson to hospital against his will, but works hard to ensure that he understands his rights and her powers within this legal framework. Matt's work with David in the Chapter 17 is grounded in his commitment to David's right to make decisions about his life, with all the work and support that that entails.

Ethical reasoning

Whilst good practice has to be anchored in law and policy, it does not follow that all practice anchored in law and policy is good. The best social work practice goes beyond immediate legal duties, so that knowing whether, when and how to intervene often involves very much more detailed and sensitive ethical judgements. Strictly speaking, if adults who have the capacity to make the decision decide to put themselves at risk, a social worker could just document this and walk away. However, a more thoughtful practitioner (like Fiona working with Ester in Chapter 12) would be asking themselves whether this person is, in reality, in the best position to make that decision. Do they know their own minds? Have they really thought about the risks? Do they need time and support to think things through? Are they just submitting to something that they do not really want? Are they frightened? The fundamental question is not so much 'is it legal?' but 'is it right?'

Jackie Pritchard describes how easy it is for social workers to 'hide behind the concept of choice' (Pritchard, 2001, p. 226), off-loading responsibility on the basis that a client has 'chosen' to drink or self-neglect or live with a violent partner. Whilst some clients are very clear about what they want to do, it may take considerable skill, time and persistence to help others to make decisions. It is often very hard to make an abstract choice – for example, whether to move into a care home – when you do not really know what any particular care home is like or how you would fit in, especially if you are filled with fear about becoming more dependent or facing the final stages of your life. In the opening section of this book, we saw how social workers often act as sources of strength and advice as well as promoters of independence and choice. Sometimes (as Nada does in the next chapter) helping someone to make a decision involves giving them the support and courage to try something different. This kind of work is based on relationships of confidence and trust, in which the social worker acts with what we earlier called 'compassionate scepticism'; 'compassionate' because there is a sense of fundamental goodwill (or unconditional positive regard) towards the client and an acknowledgment that it is, ultimately, their life and their decision, but, 'sceptical' in that a social worker may offer a different perspective and challenge the client to see their situation from other points of view.

Cultivating uncertainty

The kind of authoritative, ethical practice we are talking about here requires real skill and confidence. However, it is a confidence which arises not so much from thinking that we have great expertise (that we know everything), but from an awareness that there is so much we cannot know – a fundamental uncertainty. Ann Brechin (2000) famously describes this as a 'not-knowing' approach and it is behind much of the thinking about critical and reflective social work. Carolyn Taylor and Sue White suggest that holding on to a sense of doubt is crucial to good practice – that social workers often fall into the trap of coming to conclusions too quickly and then go on to interpret evidence in the light of their initial judgement, fitting 'the facts to the existing hypothesis' (Taylor and White, 2006, p. 950).

At first sight, uncertainty (as opposed to quick, cool decisiveness) might appear to be a rather nebulous and unsatisfactory basis for professional judgement. However, as we saw earlier, much human decision-making, whether it is by professionals or by anyone else, relies more than we would like to admit on intuitive feeling – the reactions of what Daniel Kahneman (2011) calls the 'fast-thinking' parts of our brain, whose function is to make immediate sense of a situation. Kahneman goes on to suggest that professionals can develop real expertise in making immediate decisions when the situations they encounter are relatively predicable and they have had prolonged practice in dealing with them. This might apply to a surgeon doing repeated operations or perhaps even to a social worker responding to a specific and well-defined crisis. But this kind of expertise, which relies on quickly retrieved memories of very similar past events, does not translate into contexts that play out over time and are essentially unpredictable. The danger for professionals dealing with unpredictable situations (whether they be social workers or financial traders playing the markets) is that they will be overconfident about their own knowledge:

> Paradoxically, it is easier to construct a coherent story when you know little, when there are fewer pieces to fit into the puzzle. Our comforting conviction that the world makes sense rests on a secure foundation: our almost unlimited ability to ignore our ignorance. (Kahneman, 2011, p. 201)

The need to cultivate uncertainty is not to deny that social workers have to draw on a substantial body of knowledge from a wide variety of disciplines (law, psychology, sociology and medicine to name but a few), but knowledge alone is not enough. To make good judgements in unpredictable situations, social work practice has deliberately to engage our slower-thinking and more critically reflective faculties, holding in tension different points of view (clients', carers', other professionals') alongside the perspectives of law, policy, research and rights.

Critical reflection

One of the qualities shared by all the social workers in the next three chapters (and, indeed, throughout this book) is their capacity for critical reflection – the ability to critique their own practice and to set up an almost constant internal debate. In doing so, they remain consciously and respectfully aware of the obvious (but easily forgotten) fact they are dealing with someone else's life and not their own. Where necessary, they act decisively but, even as they do so, they reflect on the consequences of their actions and use their reflections to check and modify what they are doing. Crucially, they remain alive to the ways in which they are using their influence and power and deliberately consider the sometimes painful contradictions inherent in any 'helping' relationship. We discussed earlier how promoting individual rights and encouraging 'positive risk-taking' can reduce risks and the need for protection. It is tempting, but at the same time disingenuous, to think that this can always be the case. In reality, rights and protection are sometimes in conflict:

> ...some people are dangerous, destructive, irresponsible and a risk to others or themselves, and sometimes it is necessary to limit their freedoms and try to get them to change. Very often the best practice issue is not *if* such constraint is valid, but *how* it is done in a respectful, critically reflective way which provides as much scope as possible for the service user to plan their own life. (Ferguson, 2008, p. 23)

We heard a powerful example of this kind of critically reflective debate when we interviewed a social worker (Helen) and her supervisor (Janet) about some joint work they had done with an older woman called Gwen. She was the woman we encountered briefly in the Introduction – a chronic alcoholic, whose family members took her money and used her house to drink and take drugs with their friends. Helen had tried to work with her over a period of two years but, for much of that time, she was adamant that she did not want any help, only reluctantly agreeing to accept a few visits each week from a care agency. On one particular day, the care worker found Gwen in a terrible state, sober but slumped on the floor in her own urine and faeces with severe abdominal pain. Janet and Helen visited together and, although Gwen initially turned the paramedics away, between them they persuaded her to go to hospital. From there she agreed to move into a residential home rather than return home. Her physical health improved greatly and, although she was not full of active enthusiasm for the home, she seemed to conclude that it was the lesser of two evils and decided to stay there. Helen and Janet described their feelings about what had happened:

Helen:

> [from] a purely logical point of view this is keeping somebody safe and well and giving her a longer, healthier life – it was great. But from the point of view of

her choice, we didn't really give her much choice. She was very ambivalent and it felt like a lot of persuasion was used – 'Isn't it lovely here? Haven't you got a lovely room? Aren't the staff nice?', that kind of thing... So I don't know... but I wanted her to stay there, so I had this conflict between saying to her, 'Look, you do realise what's happening to you', which I'd never have said because I didn't want her to discharge herself and go back home because then it would just be a nightmare again. So, it was a real conflict.

Janet, whilst not entirely disagreeing, had a slightly different perspective:

What I do think though is [that] statutory services too easily discharge their responsibility by saying someone has a choice. I don't agree with it – don't agree – I feel very strongly about it. I understand what Helen means... However, would I have wanted her to remain in that situation? No, I wouldn't – I'm sorry, I don't agree with it because... by statutory authorities' lack of intervention [people are] put at risk. And she was a woman who was coerced by other people into [her house] being used as a drinking den, her money used to purchase alcohol. To allow this woman to live in abject squalor for their gain. Is that right? I don't think so. And if I make a judgement on that and it's wrong, I'm sorry. But I stand by it every single time. In a sense, she acknowledged that life at home had become difficult. It had become unpleasant. She was aware that her son was taking advantage of her and she said quite clearly that she didn't want that to happen any longer. But she was somebody who did not have the physical or the mental means to stop it happening. So, do we allow that then?

Conclusion

The case studies in this final section all embody some, if not all, of the subjects we have been discussing here and illustrate the real practical and emotional difficulties that are encountered in some social work with older people. All three social workers demonstrate that their knowledge of law, policy and procedure is intrinsic to their work, a matter not just of following rules but of practising well. They show a respectful and sometimes passionate commitment to their clients' rights, which they combine with an empathetic understanding of their situations. Most of all, their work is characterised by detailed ethical reasoning – a reasoning which cultivates uncertainty by refusing to jump to easy conclusions but painstakingly and critically reflects on both the moral and practical implications of their practice.

15 Nada and Joan: Making Difficult Decisions

Questions to ask yourself as you read:

- Should social workers try to influence their clients' decisions?
- Would you have done anything differently?
- Can care homes be a positive choice or only the lesser of evils?

Nada and Joan

Joan had lived her whole life in the same small, terraced house. Born and brought up there, she had never married, had worked all her life and, since her retirement, had cared first for her parents and then for her brother until their deaths. Perhaps as a result, she had had very little opportunity to make friends and her only relative was a niece who telephoned regularly but did not live nearby. In her mid-eighties Joan had developed a number of health problems, including Parkinson's disease and, over the next three or four years, her health had deteriorated. She had started to find it more and more difficult to walk, had developed problems with swallowing and had lost a lot of weight.

Joan already had help twice a day from a care agency and regular contact with the community matron but, a few weeks before Nada met her, her doctor had asked the community-based rehabilitation service to get involved as he was becoming increasingly concerned about Joan's eating and very frequent falls. The team's remit was to provide intensive, short-term therapy at home to try to prevent hospital admissions. So, Joan had been seen by an occupational therapist, physiotherapist, community matron and speech and language therapist. They had provided some additional equipment and worked with her to try to improve her mobility and swallowing. However, there seemed to be little they could do to improve her health and they concluded that she was going to need substantially more help on a long-term basis.

Nada's first move was to meet the occupational therapist and gather as much background information as possible, from which she built up a good picture of Joan's situation. However, before she could actually visit, Joan had another fall and was admitted to hospital. Nada's first impression was of someone who had almost disappeared within this large, impersonal institution:

> It took me ages to find her because she had had two moves and she was actually lost and had ended up on the gynae ward. She had no gynae problems, it was just that there was a bed. I eventually tracked her down and she was sitting in a corner on a ward where nobody seemed to know her – the staff didn't seem to know her at all. And she's very, very tiny, so she could almost have been lost. And she was sitting there and had no visitors as her only family was a niece who lived the other side of the country.

Nada already had much of the factual information she needed for the assessment, so she was able to have a real discussion with Joan about her situation and what she wanted to do next:

> I sat and talked to her and introduced myself and asked about her and how she was. And right from the beginning she said she wanted to go home. She was determined to stay at home – absolutely. No question about that. And actually I could see that hospital was very much the wrong place for her. Because she had no family to back her up or advocate for her, she had been moved around and just wasn't getting the care and attention she needed.

There were many potential risks if Joan went home. Even with more regular visits during the day, she could still fall between times, or at night. She liked the care workers who came in to see her, but they were often late and, although she was able to take her own medication, it was difficult for her to swallow and she did so only erratically unless there was someone there with her. As a result, her Parkinson's medication was not as regular as it needed to be. And, despite input from the speech and language therapist, the care workers did not seem to have understood how important the soft diet was and had continued to give Joan things like chicken and ham cut into small pieces. Although Joan had had considerable responsibilities in her life, she was not assertive and tended to accept what other people did. So she did not protest about the food – but neither did she eat it. Even the intensive and skilled support from the rehabilitation team had not been enough to keep her out of hospital. So, Nada was very unsure how well, or for how long, Joan could be supported at home. On the other hand, having talked it through, home was where she wanted to be and it was for Joan to make the decision.

Nada's immediate role was then a very practical one. She made arrangements with the care agency and talked to them in detail about Joan's needs, particularly the importance of punctuality and the sorts of food that Joan could eat, documenting it all clearly on the care plan:

> The plan was to increase her package of care to four visits a day as soon as possible and bring her home. So that was done – assessment written up, care plan written up, the agency informed and told in no uncertain terms how critical this was.

Initially, Joan appeared reasonably well and happy. Nada went to see her after a couple of days and she was clearly pleased to be home, even though she was mostly just sitting in her chair all day. Nada felt she was very isolated, but Joan herself was unconcerned and said she did not mind being on her own. However, a week later, her health took a turn for the worse. Her niece visited her at the weekend and rang Nada to say how worried she was. Joan was, once more, not eating and the care workers were still not coming at the times agreed on the care plan:

> So I went back and she'd actually deteriorated quite markedly [and] ... I rang the GP and he came out and was very concerned.

When the doctor arrived, he and Nada checked Joan's dosette box and found that not all the tablets had been taken, which probably accounted for the deterioration. He told Joan that, in his view, she was not safe at home, but Joan said that she did not want to go anywhere. There was then nothing that Nada could do other than speak again to the care agency, which now promised they would ensure that this did not happen again. Even so, Nada continued to worry and dropped in again on her way home to check if Joan was all right. Once again, the care agency was late, so Nada stayed to give Joan her medication and make her something for tea. Before leaving, she rang the agency to double check if they were going to come and let Joan's neighbour know that Joan was not well.

Even though this visit was necessary for all the wrong reasons, Nada felt that it was something of a turning point in her relationship with Joan.

Because she was busying herself in the kitchen and doing ordinary, household tasks, they were able to have a different kind of conversation:

> While I was giving her tea, I was pottering in the kitchen and saying 'where do you keep this Joan?' and I then sat by her while she had her soup and we talked about how long she had been in the house and all her memories of growing up. And we talked about how difficult it would be to leave, but that may be something that had to happen.

The next morning, Nada was unsurprised to learn that Joan had once again been admitted to Accident and Emergency (A&E) following a fall in the night. She spoke to one of the A&E nurses who told her that Joan was not physically injured, but was very shaken and appeared so frail that they were unsure what to do.

> She was just sitting in A&E and they were wondering what to do with her. They were going to admit her, but she didn't really need to be admitted.

Nada then contacted Joan's niece, the general practitioner (GP) and the community matron to get their views. None of them thought that it would do Joan any good to be admitted to hospital: she did not need medical treatment and a hospital ward was unlikely to give her the care and attention that she did need. Instead, they agreed that Nada would talk to Joan about an immediate respite stay in a residential home to try to build up her strength and to give her time and space to make a plan for the longer term.

This time, Joan accepted the suggested respite, even though the only room that Nada could find at short notice was in a residential home some way outside her home town. Nada spoke to the home manager, who agreed to come two or three hours later and, much to Nada's relief and pleasure, she instantly struck up a good rapport with Joan:

> So I went down to A&E with the care home manager... and it was great. They clicked. They got on really well, really well. And it was fantastic. They were funny as well – I think I'd been quite serious, but they came in, making jokes, you know, which she really responded to. And she was beaming away and I thought 'this is great'.

Joan had nothing to take with her, so whilst she went to the residential home, Nada collected her things:

> Of course she had no clothes, no medication. So I phoned the Community Matron [as] I couldn't go into the house on my own and pack a suitcase. So we

*had to go through her cupboards and try to work out [what] she would need.
And I took it down to the home and made sure the house was locked up and
told the neighbour where she was.*

As so often, Nada's memory of the human story is much clearer than
her memory of the administrative processes she had to go through:

*I can't remember how funding was agreed, but somewhere along the line, it
was [laughing]. I think it might have been agreed retrospectively.*

Joan got on very well at the residential home and being 'looked after'
seemed, almost immediately, to have a positive effect:

*Within a week, she'd turned around. She responded really well to all the TLC
[tender loving care]. She was eating, walking around. I saw her walk from her
bedroom to the dining room on her own, sat down, huge roast dinner, tucked
in, no problems, smiling – really, really responded well.*

The next stage was then to talk to Joan about the future. There was no
question of Joan's capacity to decide where she should live, but Nada
felt that she was not very realistic about her situation:

*Somehow, although she certainly had capacity to make the decision about
where she should live, it seemed that she hadn't quite caught up with her
recent deterioration in terms of her mobility. She did recall the falls, but mini-
mised them really – 'I can manage, it doesn't matter'.*

Joan was very unsure what to do next. On the one hand, she still
wanted to go home and felt that she would be able to manage now that
she was better. But, she was also very keen to know what her family,
Nada and her doctor all thought about it. Nada's opinion (shared by
the GP and the community matron) was that Joan was 'better' because
of the continual care and attention she was now receiving and that,
if she went back home, she would almost certainly have further falls
and her health would deteriorate again. Changes and improvements
in her care arrangements might help but, in reality, it is all too usual
for busy care workers to be late. Even if they were more reliable, there
would still be significant risks to Joan between care visits and she was
very isolated. It seemed that what had really helped was to have people
around all the time, partly for company and partly so that there was
someone 'on hand' as and when Joan needed them. The amount of
funding that the local authority would contribute would not be enough
to pay for a live-in carer. In any case, Joan did not have a spare room

and, as she often needed help at night, it might have been too much for one person. Nada looked into the possibility of an 'extra care' flat, but Joan's needs were considered too high. Joan's family were very clear about what they thought:

> The family were all saying 'you're not going to move her home, are you?' But that's what she wanted, to move back to her house. And she was saying 'I'm alright now', but I knew that she was alright because of all the continual attention and care that she was getting. That was a really difficult one.

Nada visited Joan on a number of occasions over a period of a few weeks and they discussed the risks of going home and the potential positives and negatives of staying in residential care. They identified what was really important to Joan, like living in her home town and having her own things around her and talked about how this might be done.

> I felt I had to allow her to come to a decision – almost to come to an agreement – with as much of what she wanted in that outcome as possible. And I think there was also a lot of acknowledgement that it was a huge event for her – a huge, life-changing event for her. Something enormous for her to consider. And the acknowledgement of that – it wasn't just riding roughshod over her feelings.

Eventually, Joan decided that she would try moving into a residential home near to her house. She knew someone who had gone to live there and had heard good things about it from others. The manager came to see her and, as luck would have it, a room became available quite quickly and Joan was able to move in. She continued to miss her own home, but appreciated the comfort and company in residential care. It was not what she had wanted, but she seemed to feel it had been the right decision.

Discussion

Joan's story is likely to resonate with most social workers working with older people, exposing, as it does, both the inadequacies of parts of the care system and the real vulnerability which can accompany age and ill health. Many older people move into care homes following some sort of crisis, often involving an admission to hospital. Frequent falls are often a contributory factor, as are isolation, low morale and loss of confidence (Taylor and Donnelly, 2006). We cannot know whether, if the home care Joan received had been better, she could have remained at home a bit longer or whether her health was simply too unstable and her needs too high. But the reality was that the service she received was far from perfect and this may well have been one of the factors that contributed to her move into residential care. Nada did what she could by writing detailed care plans, repeatedly talking to the agency and feeding back her concerns, but she could not actually control what happened day by day. Maureen Eby talks about social workers, whilst holding on to ideals, having to be 'utterly realistic about the constraints that exist in any organisational, and indeed personal, context' (Eby, 2000, p. 118). In helping Joan to make decisions about long-term care arrangements, Nada had to be realistic and work with the options that were actually there.

From the start, Nada was deeply respectful in the way she worked. When she first saw Joan in hospital, she was very aware of her vulnerability and the high risk that she would come to harm if she returned home. But she also spent time talking to Joan, finding out about her life and the things that were important for her. She recognised her strengths and avoided simply defining Joan in her own mind as frail, at risk, and in need of protection:

> *She had worked all her life in the public sector. She was very independent – self-sufficient actually – quite used to living alone.*

She also allowed time for Joan to make her own decisions which, initially, involved supporting her to go home. Nada herself thought it was likely that this would not work out, or at least would not work out for long, but she recognised that it was something Joan had to try – and that it was her right to do so. When Joan had her second fall, Nada prevented her hospital admission, which might well have led to Joan having to make a rushed decisions about her care when she was discharged. Instead, Nada negotiated a short stay in a residential home – a period of stability in which Joan could think about her future. She consciously and explicitly made 'temporary' arrangements so that Joan did not have to burn her boats by, for example, selling her house, before she had come to a decision.

Although there is much talk of 'risk' in social work, the word 'uncertainty' better captures the sense that many aspects of the work are essentially unpredictable (Macdonald and Macdonald, 2010). Being uncertain is uncomfortable precisely because it cannot be measured or 'managed' and the temptation for social workers is to try to resolve things as quickly as possible, particularly when someone might be harmed. But, if people are rushed, they may feel pushed into something that they never wanted to happen, which will harm them in a different way. On the other hand, staying uncertain, or at least avoiding dogmatic certainty, does not mean that social workers should not use their knowledge and experience to develop an informed view. Nada had seen at first hand how quickly Joan's health deteriorated if anything went even slightly wrong. Although she wanted to be at home, in many ways her quality of life there was poor. Her health had dramatically improved in residential care and she had enjoyed the company. Objectively, it would have been difficult for Nada not to think that this was the better option, especially as Joan's family and her doctor agreed.

What was very clear listening to Nada was that she cared about Joan. She knew it was Joan's right to make decisions but she also did not want her to come to harm – there was an ethical as well as a legal dimension to her work. Richard Sennett (2003) writes about the way in which 'dependency' on each other is fundamental to private, personal relationships, but is perceived as almost shameful in the public sphere. Something rather similar is going on with the idea of 'protection'. In our personal lives, wanting to protect people close to us is seen as perfectly natural. In fact, not wanting to protect them would appear hard-hearted and neglectful. But in the public world of social care, 'protection' is inherently suspect. There is too long a history of damage done by often well-intentioned intervention in people's lives for it to be otherwise. What can be very troubling to social workers is that the relationship we have with our clients, though professional, can also feel very personal, intimately involved as we sometimes are in people's lives. In fact, we have been arguing throughout this book that genuine relationships are at the heart of good social work practice and we often care about the people we work with. And yet we also know how suffocating, and sometimes dangerous, 'protection' can be.

On the day Nada found Joan in bed, she went back to see her after work because she did not want her to come to any harm. But, she was also acutely aware of the tensions in her position, showing the kind of reflective, critical thinking that characterises good practice. As she talked to Joan in A&E about the idea of respite, Joan wanted to know what her niece thought she should do. Nada told her, but also worried that, in doing so, she was exerting too much influence and 'persuading' Joan to accept the residential home:

> Feeling very manipulative, I said that I had spoken to her niece and her husband, because she was very interested in what they wanted... and she thought it was a really good idea that she went.

Similarly, when Joan agreed to the respite, Nada felt uncomfortable and questioned whether she was doing the right thing. She was absolutely clear that the arrangement she was making with the residential home was a temporary one and that Joan had every right to decide to return home. But she also thought that, if Joan had this respite break it was, in reality, less likely that she would go home again:

> So I actually felt like I was betraying her at that point, because I knew that if she went to the care home for six weeks respite, she probably wasn't going to go home. So I felt very uncomfortable about that. However, she was agreeing to go there.

Sandra Dwyer (2005) suggests that it is often relatives who arrange for older people to move into care homes and the views of the older persons themselves can easily be overlooked. Nada showed herself to be very aware of this in the way she reflected on and critiqued her own practice. But, what made it more difficult was that Joan herself seemed to value the opinions of others (her family, her doctor and Nada) almost above her own. It was almost as if she wanted the decision taken out of her hands.

> It was very, very difficult actually. And what made it even more difficult was that she was quite passive – not passive, but she didn't disagree. In a way it was almost as if I was the authority figure, especially with the weight of all these [other people's opinions] I was bringing into the room with me.

Perhaps Joan's decision-making also calls into question the usefulness of a rather 'thin' conception of individual choice as something that happens in isolation – simply the exercise of my will or my right. Joan was not simply asserting her wish to live at home as opposed to her family's view that she would not be safe. It was more that the views of her family and of the professionals involved were important to her and formed part of her decision making. When people make decisions, they do so as 'thickly constituted, morally encumbered selves' (Sandel, 2010, p. 248): in other words, as people whose histories, beliefs, personalities and relationships are woven into their sense of who they are:

> When confronted with competing paths, I try to figure out which path will best make sense of my life as a whole, and of the things I care about. Moral deliberation is more about interpreting my life story than exerting my will. (Sandel, 2010, p. 221)

Nada's work illustrates the endless dilemmas of social work – the inevitability of compromise and virtual impossibility of getting things objectively right, because there is no clear, objective 'right' out there. She worked within the law in being clear that any decision was for Joan herself to make. Her attitude was respectful, working with Joan in coming to decisions whilst acting with 'compassionate scepticism', using her experience and knowledge to question Joan's perception of her needs. And yet, in so doing, she clearly used her position and authority to influence Joan and the final decision that she made. In the end, it is not possible to draw a hard and fast line between legitimate influence on the one hand and persuasion on the other. Fiona, in Chapter 12, worries that she has not done enough to try to persuade Ester to accept residential care and has left her at risk. Nada worries that she has been too persuasive. However, Nada's skill throughout this work was underpinned by the way she acknowledged this and kept up a reflexive debate, using the tensions to question, check and modify her own practice.

16

Jane and Mr Wilson: Using Legal Powers

Questions to ask yourself as you read:

- Why is multi-disciplinary working so important in this kind of situation?
- How can intervening in a person's life against their will be positive?
- If Mr Wilson had refused to move from hospital into a care home, what would Jane's options have been?

Jane and Mr Wilson

Jane's work with Mr Wilson is, in some respects, different from the other practices we have looked at in this book as it takes place within the formal procedural and legal frameworks of Safeguarding Adults and the Mental Capacity Act 2005 (MCA). At the point when Jane was allocated the case, a Safeguarding referral had already been made by the care agency as they had concerns about Mr Wilson's care and the management of his money. Jane's initial remit was to attend a multi-disciplinary 'strategy meeting' with the agency, general practitioner (GP), district nurse and occupational therapist in order to share information and agree how best to approach the situation.

Strategy meeting

Listening to the different professionals at the meeting, Jane began to build up a picture. Mr Wilson had run his own business until his mid-sixties when he had had a stroke, which left him with impaired mobility. Now in his nineties, he had become almost immobile and something of a recluse, living upstairs in an increasingly neglected cottage, which he had not been out of for years. The care agency had not found him easy to work with. He would often tell them that he did not want any help and send them away, only then to complain that he had been neglected, and he could be both rude and sexually inappropriate. The agency was worried that they would end up not having enough care workers who were willing to support him.

Two or three weeks before the meeting Mr Wilson had had a fall, which further reduced his mobility so that he was no longer able to get to his bathroom. The community rehabilitation team had been working with him since the fall, but had found him either reluctant to accept their advice or unable to take it in. He insisted that he could still get out of bed with minimal assistance, whilst in reality he needed very considerable help. He also refused to have any equipment, so supporting him while he transferred would have put the care workers at serious risk of injuring themselves. As a result, he was spending all the time in bed and, unable to get out to use the commode, was trying to manage with a bowl. He often refused help from the care workers, insisting that he could cope or saying that they needed to come back later. The district nurse had real concerns about his skin care as he could easily develop pressure sores, but again he said that he did not want a hospital bed or any pressure-relieving mattress.

Sometimes he seemed forgetful. After one occupational therapy session, he had asked to be left in a particular chair until the next visit, but had then made a series of panicky phone calls to say that he had been abandoned. At the same time, he was very articulate and, in many ways, astute. Any kind of discussion was difficult as he would talk continuously, repeatedly expressing his point of view, going off on a tangent and deflecting any attempts by others to give their opinions:

> In his own home he made it very difficult, however skilled you were. He was very much in charge, he was very articulate and he was very keen to explain things in the way that he wanted – really to dominate the conversation. To actually interrupt or to say 'we're not here to talk about that and we really need to focus on this' was well-nigh impossible... He would say, 'No, no, you need to listen while I tell you this.'

When the occupational therapist tried to discuss some of the problems with him, he became very angry, maintaining that she had not allowed him to try to get himself out of bed and in no way acknowledging that many attempts had been made to help him, but that he had not been able to do it:

> *[The occupational therapist] said she spent two hours one Sunday morning, with him [insisting] 'I can do it this way'. In the end she said to him 'well, you show me how you think you could do it'. And it was how he used to do it, but he couldn't do it now. That was a major cause of dispute, that they hadn't let him do it, that they hadn't let him sit in the chair that he liked to sit in. But, in fact, he didn't ever really acknowledge that they had tried – and failed, because of his deterioration.*

To add to the complications, Mr Wilson had a friend, a much younger woman called Tanya, who visited him regularly and did some shopping, cleaning and cooking. He was very fond of her and, when the care workers offered him something for lunch or tea, he would often say he did not need it as Tanya would be calling later. However, as she did not come every day, and was sometimes away for periods of time, he often had nothing to eat or drink. The care agency had also become aware that Tanya used Mr Wilson's bank card and he made references to the fact that he had given her money.

At the end of the meeting, a number of decisions were made. Jane and the district nurse would review Mr Wilson's care to look at the issues with him once again and see if they could be resolved. Jane would also talk to Tanya to clarify what support she was providing and what access she had to Mr Wilson's money. The other major consideration was whether Mr Wilson had the capacity to decide what care he received and who he gave his money to. It was agreed that, as this was likely to be a complex assessment and major decisions might need to be made, Mr Wilson's GP would talk to him about a referral to a geriatrician who could provide some specialist expertise in relation to his mental health.

Safeguarding assessment

After the strategy meeting, Jane arranged to visit Mr Wilson with his friend Tanya and the district nurse. Jane explained that the professionals involved all agreed that he needed two care workers with appropriate equipment to help him get out of bed and that, with that provision, they believed that he could be supported at home. However, Mr Wilson remained adamant that he did not want any changes made as he felt sure he would soon improve and be able to walk again.

During the course of this meeting, Jane also started to assess Mr Wilson's mental capacity to make decisions about his care and finances. The MCA Code of Practice (Great Britain, Department for Constitutional Affairs, 2007) is clear that people should not be labelled as lacking capacity simply because they are making an unwise decision. There was no question that Mr Wilson was able to understand and retain information and communicate his own views and it was quite possible that his somewhat obstinate refusal to listen to anyone else was simply part of his character. And yet, it appeared to Jane that there was more to it than this:

> It was very tricky. I thought probably he had good understanding of his immediate situation but he lacked insight into the implications of the decisions he was making... so though he could say 'Tanya will be in later so it doesn't matter if I don't eat now', his ability to think 'well what do I do if she doesn't come in and what are the implications of that... it was all that side of it.... It was his lack of judgement really.

When the geriatrician visited, he was of the same mind and concluded that Mr Wilson lacked the capacity to make decisions about his future care or his finances. On the one hand, he appeared to be very clear about what he wanted (or did not want) and he scored high in a memory test. However, he did not seem able to weigh up information he was given; he could not say what his care needs were or think about the future, maintaining that there were no real problems. Significantly, he was later diagnosed with fronto-temporal dementia, the symptoms of which can include a lack of insight and empathy, inappropriate behaviour, loss of inhibition and circumlocution in speech (Alzheimers Society, 2010).

In relation to his money, it was true that Tanya had Mr Wilson's bank card and sometimes used his money to buy things for herself. However, Mr Wilson said he was happy with this arrangement. He was very fond of her, she helped him and he wanted to give her something for it.

> She had been using his debit card for her own shopping. But he had said he wanted her to do that. That was the trouble. She kept saying to me 'he wants me to – he wants me to take a taxi if I'm tired'. And he would say the same thing.

This arrangement had been going on for several years and, although Tanya profited from it, it had also benefited Mr Wilson. Looking back on previous records, it was evident that other young women had helped Mr Wilson in the past and he had also given them money – at a time when he did have capacity to make this decision. Jane knew that, according to the MCA Code of Practice, she needed to take his past wishes and feelings into account in any decisions about his money. At the same time, the arrangement did leave Mr Wilson exposed to considerable financial risk. Jane discussed this with Tanya and explained the risks both to her and to Mr Wilson of her holding his bank card without any sort of authority. Although Mr Wilson lacked capacity to make decisions about his finances as a whole, he would have liked Tanya to have managed them on his behalf. However, Tanya said that she did not want a formal role for herself as it would involve too much responsibility and paperwork.

Best interests decisions and safeguarding plan

It was now clear that 'best interests decisions' needed to be made in relation to Mr Wilson's care and finances. He had no family and, following Safeguarding guidance, Jane referred him to the local Independent Mental Capacity Advocate (IMCA) service so that he could be properly represented during this process.

In relation to his finances, one option was for the local authority to apply to the Court of Protection for Deputyship, but they would not do this unless Mr Wilson became a permanent resident in a care home. So a decision could not be made until his future care arrangements were clear. In the meantime, Jane advised Tanya that she needed to be very careful about how she used his funds, as this would be scrutinised by any future Deputy. Decisions about Mr Wilson's care were even more difficult. Mr Wilson had clearly stated that he did not want more care at home or to move into a nursing home, so it seemed likely that both of these options would cause him considerable distress. After further discussions, it was agreed that Jane and the IMCA would speak to him about the less restrictive option of going to hospital for a period of intensive rehabilitation and treatment, to see whether his health and mobility could be improved. If it could, it might then be possible for him to return home without the need for equipment.

> So I went back with the IMCA because what we then went on to suggest [was] that, because he was refusing admission to a nursing home... how would he feel about going into hospital? And he said that he didn't want to consider that either. He did say that he needed a course of treatment... but he didn't need to be [in hospital] to have it.

It felt as if they were going round in circles and, at the same time, Mr Wilson's situation was worsening as he spent more days at home, in bed without adequate care. So, in close consultation with Mr Wilson's GP, the geriatrician, district nurse, ambulance service, Jane's manager and the legal department, agreement was reached that he should be admitted to hospital even if he did not agree. This could happen within the main MCA Code of Practice provided Mr Wilson was not restricted or restrained. If restraints or restrictions did have to be imposed, the hospital would need to consider whether it might constitute a 'deprivation of liberty'. If so, they would have to apply for authorisation under the Deprivation of Liberty Safeguards (Great Britain, Ministry of Justice, 2008).

Jane and the district nurse went to see Mr Wilson again to explain this to him and the GP arranged for an ambulance to collect him later that day, reasoning that giving him more notice than this would be unlikely to achieve anything, but could cause him considerable anxiety. Jane started by explaining the 'best interests' decision again and the legal context in which this was made:

> [I] said that we really felt that he should go into hospital...[and] that, if we could get him home, we would – that this genuinely was a period ideally of rehabilitation and we would be working towards getting him home.

Their hope was that Mr Wilson would finally agree, but he was unyielding:

> We had a really very demanding couple of hours with him as he would not give way and he was very articulate as to what his objections were. When the paramedics arrived, he continued to say no. He said 'you can't take me without a judge saying so'...I'd actually printed off the [relevant sections of the MCA Code of Practice] and one of the paramedics ended up reading it out to him. And he did say he needed to talk to his solicitor and we said 'well fine, talk to your solicitor', but you know he then said – 'I'm not going to pay him'.

So, at last, whilst still not actively agreeing, Mr Wilson did not protest about being taken to hospital and the paramedics were able to lift him into the ambulance and transport him without using any restraint. Jane and the district nurse went with him and, to their surprise and relief, once he was there, he did not object at all. He settled down on the ward, accepted the treatment and care he was given and did not ask to go home.

Review

Mr Wilson was in hospital for three or four weeks for treatment and further rehabilitation, but it was to no avail:

> What they had tried to do during the time was get him back on his feet, [but] he couldn't. He was too anxious so they couldn't even really stand him.

During this time, Tanya had made it clear that she could not offer him any help with his personal care and had also told him that she had to go away for a few weeks, so would not be able to support him if he returned home immediately. (At Jane's request, she also agreed to leave Mr Wilson's bank card behind.) The care agency said that they did not want to restart the package as there were so few care workers now who would work with him. Thinking again about his best interests, it seemed very unlikely that his needs could be met at home. When Jane and the hospital doctor (and later the IMCA) talked to him about what should happen next, to their surprise, he agreed to move into a nursing home, at least while Tanya was away:

> He did say that one of the difficulties for him in receiving care at home was getting the care staff he wants for the time he needed them. So, I felt that he was showing a little bit of recognition of the fact that in hospital it had been very much easier [for him to receive] the care that he needed.

It turned out better than anyone could have predicted. When Jane first went to see him after he had moved, Mr Wilson was glowing in his praise for the home:

> He said the care he was receiving was 'inexpressively good. Nothing else could improve his stay'. He thanked the chef for the lovely food. He would like to take communion. It really was amazing... He said he thought things should remain as they are though he was looking forward to [when] his friend Tanya would be returning and taking charge of his care arrangements again.

He struck up an immediate rapport with one of the nurses and agreed to use a hospital bed with pressure-relieving mattress. He accepted care from two members of staff during the day and frequently at night, his skin was in good condition and he was able to eat and drink more independently than before as he could be positioned better in bed.

When Tanya returned, Jane reviewed the situation again, talking to her and Mr Wilson together and on their own on several occasions.

Both of them seemed unsure about the future. Sometimes Tanya would say that she would move in with Mr Wilson if he went home, but she would also say that she did not want to manage his money on a formal basis and could not provide any personal care because of her own poor health. Jane would then talk to her about the amount of care that he needed during the day and at night, at which point she would hesitate again. Mr Wilson was also inconsistent. When he had just seen Tanya, he would sometimes get distressed and say that he wanted to go home with her, but most of the time, it seemed that he wanted to stay:

> He had started to say that maybe the house would have to be sold... He'd asked nurse to come and see him and said to him that it didn't look as if he would be able to go home because there was no one to look after him and he'd asked if he could stay on at the home.

It was almost as if this state of suspended decision-making suited them. They were able to talk to each other as if maybe, one day, if things were different they could be together and to keep that idea alive without actually committing themselves to it.

Jane began to consider whether social services would need to apply to the Court of Protection both to manage Mr Wilson's finances and resolve the question of whether it was in his best interests to remain permanently at the care home. But, just a few days after one of the meetings, Mr Wilson developed a chest infection, was admitted to hospital and died. It was very sudden, but in many ways Jane felt that it spared him – that it was better that he did not have to cope with the decisions that would have had to follow:

> I think probably it was a good outcome because he died before he had to make any final, difficult decisions or we had to tell him that that was the decision that would have to be made. [I don't mean it] in a heartless way... I think in a way that's what you feel with your own parents and friends as well. That's what you want, or at least what I want, is that it's timely and that it's a good outcome, you know. There are similarities in how you feel – that it was for the best.

Discussion

Reading about Jane's work with Mr Wilson, it is striking how many different but overlapping processes and frameworks she had to work with – never mind the complexities of the human situation. There was the overarching framework of the Safeguarding Adults procedure with its strategy meetings and safeguarding assessments, plans and reviews. Within this, she was reviewing Mr Wilson's care and securing funding for a placement within the usual community care processes whilst, at the same time, working with the legal requirements of the Mental Capacity Act 2005 to complete a mental capacity assessment and make 'best interests' decisions. Although, in common with all the social workers we spoke to, she focussed on the human rather than the procedural story; all these processes would have had different paperwork, guidance and timescales.

The legal aspects of the work are complex – involving fine judgements about capacity, restriction and best interests. Jane's skill reveals itself in the way in which, whilst she very explicitly follows legislation and guidance, they seem to be intrinsic to her practice rather than dictating from the outside the way in which she works. For example, she takes a highly collaborative approach, working closely with health colleagues, particularly when difficult decisions have to be made. She involves Mr Wilson every step of the way, trying to negotiate solutions that will be acceptable to him and taking his views seriously even when they had to be overruled. But there is a sense in which she is not doing this in order to follow Safeguarding guidance and the MCA Code (although she is doing so), but because it is good, defensible practice. Perhaps this is partly the 'unconscious competence' of an experienced social worker, but it also seems to demonstrate a high degree of ethical reasoning, a deep-seated seriousness and respect for her client. As Stephen Webb says:

> The social worker has an ethical disposition to do the best for clients. ... This is not about adherence to duty-bound rules or a set of prescribed codes of conduct. That is conformity. Practising values and believing in them are acts of an ethical disposition or will. (Webb, 2006, p. 203)

We can look at this in the detailed judgements Jane made about where and how to intervene, establishing the boundaries of her own involvement and influence. At the initial strategy meeting, there was some discussion about Mr Wilson's relationship with Tanya – the fact that she was a much younger woman and that he had given her substantial sums of money. Views were expressed that the relationship was inappropriate, that Tanya was 'grooming' and exploiting Mr Wilson, using his affection to get money. Kate Spreadbury, in her analysis of her role chairing often highly charged Safeguarding Adults meetings (Jones and Spreadbury, 2008, p. 187), writes about the dangers of professionals coming to conclusions too quickly, constructing a particular 'taken for granted discourse' before a thorough assessment has taken place. Jane also felt that they were leaping to conclusions and consciously kept an open mind, what Ann Brechin calls a 'not-knowing approach' (Brechin, 2000, p. 32). Through talking to Mr Wilson and Tanya, she came to understand that their relationship was meaningful to both of them:

> *He did view her probably as a kind of granddaughter. That was how she viewed the relationship, she said. But she also said she sometimes wondered whether he was a bit in love with her... He said things like 'she's my angel and I couldn't imagine life without her'. I think it did give them both pleasure. She was very kind to him [and] would spend a lot of time there.*

Jane also saw the financial arrangement in the context of a history in which Mr Wilson (when he still had capacity to make the decision) had chosen to give money away to other young women who had cared for him. It may not have been wise and some may have viewed it as 'inappropriate', but in Jane's analysis, neither of these were really her business:

> *I didn't feel that either of them was doing anything that the other one didn't want to happen. He did give her quite a lot of money. But, I just thought – I don't know – if it makes them happy... because when their relationship started, he did have the capacity to make these decisions.*

Rather than relying on broad principles (older man + younger woman + substantial amounts of money = abuse), this kind of 'narrative' ethical reasoning emerges out of a commitment to understanding the often complex detail of individual relationships and emotions (Banks, 2008). It demands that, to practise well, social workers need to pay close attention to the individual and never lose sight of their 'face' (Frank, 2004). At the strategy meeting, Jane could have framed Tanya's involvement in the language of 'abuse' and pursued it accordingly, involving the police and trying immediately to stop her accessing Mr Wilson's funds. This might have saved him some money but could also have destroyed his friendship. It would have been committing a kind of violence:

> *... the violence of telling people that they should not be who they are, or that they fail to understand who they ought to be.* (Frank, 2004, p. 115)

Jane decided instead to work with Tanya, explaining to her the need for a more formal financial arrangement and advising her that, for her own sake as well as his, she should be careful how she used his money from now on.

Jane was also careful about the way in which she worked with Mr Wilson. Throughout this book, we have been arguing that relationship is central to good social work practice. But, relationships can take many forms. In this situation, Jane felt it was important that she maintained a professional detachment, addressing him throughout by his title and surname:

I had a certain amount of respect for him and listened to what he said but I did keep a certain distance and think he probably was aware of that.

She realised that, for Mr Wilson, the boundaries between professional concern and friendship were quite blurred, which, perhaps, explains his inappropriate behaviour with some of his care workers. He would often ring his doctor for a chat and, after he had been seen by the geriatrician, felt betrayed by his conclusions, as he had understood that he was coming to see him as a friend and had talked to him as such. It was therefore necessary for her, in exercising her legal powers, to be very clear about her role so that he knew where he stood.

So, whilst Jane paid close attention to Mr Wilson's point of view, she did not get drawn into it. She was able to take a step back and analyse the bigger picture, identifying the points at which his opinions could not necessarily prevail and considering objectively the effects of dementia on his behaviour. We discussed in Chapter 14 how an uncritical emphasis on individual rights and choice can make almost any sort of intervention seem like interference. As a result, social workers may feel they have no right to intervene and (often with a sigh of relief) conclude that they have no further responsibility as their client is choosing to put themselves at risk. There will always be profound ethical dilemmas when social workers make judgements about other people's lives, and it is perhaps inevitable that this sort of decision will be morally compromised. Jane, and the other professionals she worked with, tried hard to negotiate with Mr Wilson, but ultimately decided to use the legal powers which they had to intervene against his will. It was always going to be a risk – they could not have known that Mr Wilson would actually like being in hospital and enjoy the nursing home. But it was a positive kind of risk-taking, not simply trying to prevent harm, but aiming to progress and improve Mr Wilson's life.

17 Matt and David: Positive Risk-Taking

Questions to ask yourself as you read:

- What do you think David's father might have been thinking?
- How can you tell the difference between agreement and compliance?
- If you had been David's social worker, would you have done anything differently?

Matt and David

Matt had no idea what to expect when he first arrived at David's house as, despite David's age and disability, he had never had any contact with social services. All Matt knew was that David was in his mid-sixties, had been deaf since birth and had lived with his parents all his life. His mother had recently died and his father was very frail, so the family had had some recent contact with their general practitioner (GP). It was the district nurse who had made the referral, concerned that David's father was no longer able to look after him.

Matt was asked to do the assessment because he was part of a specialist team and was fluent in British Sign Language (BSL). However, when he first tried to communicate with David, he found that he was unable to take part in any sort of conversation. He was profoundly deaf, his lip reading was very limited, he knew no BSL and relied almost entirely on gesture and guesswork:

> At home he relied on clues like names he could lip read, or clues from people's behaviour – Mum going into the kitchen [means it's] dinner time, or putting a coat on [means we're] going out. Just basic clues.

Talking to David's father and his sister, Margaret, Matt learned that David had been thrown out of a school for deaf children as a young teenager because of his behaviour and had never finished his education. Neither his parents nor his sister could sign, so he had never developed a proper first language. He had lived at home all his life, with virtually no social contact and no means of communication.

> *It wasn't clear to me whether he had learning difficulties. But, from my knowledge of the Deaf world, I was inclined to assume that he didn't, but that he had massive gaps in his learning because of his [life experiences].*

David's father did not want any involvement with the 'authorities' and, although he let Matt in, was both reluctant and defensive. However, David's sister was more open, realising that, once their father died, David was going to need considerable support. As for David himself, Matt had no immediate way of finding out what he wanted or thought about anything:

> *I didn't really know what I was going to do with this case at all. I felt quite a mixture of feelings. I felt quite angry with the family. I couldn't show it, but inside I was thinking 'how could you deprive this man of a life?'. But then also quite excited about – well now's his opportunity to get out and see some of the world.*

Discussing his visit and initial assessment in supervision, it was clear that Matt was going to have to spend considerable time with David in order to complete an assessment, work out what kind of support he would need and plan his future. It was agreed that he would start by visiting weekly and would use this time to build up a relationship and find a way of communicating. Never having encountered a situation quite like this before, there was an element of improvisation:

> *When I [first] went in, I thought 'what am I going to do? How are we going to spend the time?' So I'd arrive at the house and his father would say 'he's in there' and shut the door and go and have a snooze. So I had an hour with David. I used to take in library books, magazines, pens and paper and things like that and just do some activities. Partly to try to find out whether he had any signing and literacy skills and partly just as something fun to do.*

It quickly became clear to Matt that David was very keen to learn. He seemed to enjoy the visits and started to memorise the signs for some of the things in the picture books they looked at. However, David's father continued to treat Matt with suspicion and a degree of hostility:

It wasn't easy going in there because I knew his father didn't want me there. But that made me feel that it was more important for me to get in there and advocate for [David]. Or at least to find out from him whether he wanted something more from life.

David had never been allowed out on his own, even in his local area, so Matt had no way of knowing what his vision was like, whether he could cross a road safely or how confident he would be outside. The opportunity came one day when the family had run out of milk. Matt offered to go and get some and asked if he could take David with him, to which his father agreed. David seemed very much to know what he was doing, taking the key and locking the door unprompted, showing Matt the way to the corner shop and making a beeline for the fridge where the milk was on sale. For the next few weeks, going out became part of the routine and Matt was able to build up a much more detailed picture of David's skills.

And then, quite suddenly, David's father was admitted to hospital and died. David had immediately to move in with his sister, who lived on her own in a house nearby. This was workable in the very short term, but Margaret suffered from depression and had other health problems and she was clear that she could not look after her brother. As an interim measure, Matt arranged for David to start at a local workshop for deaf people, partly to see how he would get on socially and partly to give his sister a regular break ('He absolutely loved it. He was just so, so keen.'). However, with Margaret under increasing stress, there was pressure to agree a long-term plan with David. Margaret wanted him to move as soon as possible, but Matt felt strongly that they needed to find a placement where David could continue to develop his skills and independence:

I was under a lot of pressure to find a placement for him fairly quickly, which for someone who is deaf and not having any of the life skills [was not easy]. He was very fit health-wise and just wouldn't have fitted into [an older people's care home]. ... it needed to be something quite specific for him.

Very fortunately, a couple of months later, a vacancy did come up in a shared 'supported-living' house, which could offer 24-hour support and had staff who could sign. Confident by now that David did not have a learning difficulty and encouraged by his obvious eagerness to learn, Matt felt sure that David would develop the skills he needed to live more independently in the future. Margaret, however, was less certain:

We visited and [Margaret] had reservations, because she had in her mind the idea of a group home – something more old-fashioned and protected.

There was another major hurdle. The supported living option was expensive and Matt's senior managers were concerned that, if David did not acquire more independent living skills, social services would be committed to this level of funding for years to come. Matt felt immensely frustrated by the hoops he had to jump through to get the funding approved. Part of his frustration was a sense that his professional judgement was being undermined. With such a painstaking, hands-on assessment over a considerable length of time, he had by now a very good idea of what would and what would not work for David. But this was being called into question by people who had never even met him:

> Then we had to go to the Panel [meeting to agree funding]. That was horrendous really because they kept coming back to me and saying 'Well have you thought about this option?' because [the supported living] was expensive. So I then had to go and visit inappropriate places and evidence the fact that we had looked at every other option and why it wasn't appropriate. It was a waste of time – visiting other homes, phoning round, having to write lengthy reports about why places weren't appropriate, when I had found a place that was appropriate. I think that's really difficult, because you use your skills to find an appropriate service for somebody, but it's not accepted, your skills are [dismissed] really... I'd spent months working with him in a one-to-one way to get to know him and find out what was really going to be right for him.

More fundamentally, Matt felt passionately that David had missed out on so much, it would be a terrible injustice if he were now not given a chance to develop and have a life of his own. His parents had been so protective of him that he had never done anything outside his home and, until now, he had been completely ignored or failed by statutory services. He had never developed any interests, never had any friends, never decided for himself what to eat, never been away or chosen his own clothes, never been swimming and never been to the cinema:

> This man had had nothing – no services for the whole of his life. He didn't have education, no further education. You know, I think that [if he] had had a different upbringing he probably would have had a family, a job, his own home, probably a partner. His life would have been so different. So I felt we owed it to him to find him the best place that would give him a future. Although he was in his 60's, to me it's never too late. He can have a good quality of live. He could live until he's 100, you know. Or even if it's only ten years – if we can give him the best ten years of his life, then he deserves

that. Because I think someone should have been in there [earlier in his life] advocating for him.

Matt particularly felt that he had to act as an advocate because, quite apart from his communication difficulties, David was easy-going by tempera-ment and, having had so little experience, did not have the knowledge that he needed to state a preference or make choices. It would have been all too easy to have moved him into a care home where he probably would have been content to stay, because he knew of nothing else:

Because he was easy, he was happy to watch films on TV and look at picture books, he was no trouble. And I think because of that it would have been very easy to have just written him off. It's quite often the service users who are challenging – they're the ones [social services will] spend a lot of time and money on.

Eventually, Matt won his argument and funding was agreed for up to three years. Supporting David to move was the next challenge, as Matt could not simply explain the situation or ask David if he wanted to go.

I did a lot of work with him around moving in, trying to prepare him for that – taking photographs of him in the room, buying things for the room, putting his name and photograph on the bedroom door – left a couple of things in the room that were his, so that he could get the idea that this was where he was going to go. Because we couldn't explain that to him. We couldn't ask him if that was where he wanted to go.

When David did move it was an instant success:

He settled in wonderfully. He absolutely loved it... He was beginning to learn some basic sign language – he picked things up so quickly... He went from strength to strength really.

It was, however, difficult for Margaret. As she saw David starting to thrive, she could not help but realise how limited his life had been. Matt tried to keep her involved, but as David started to communicate using some basic BSL, Margaret felt all the more excluded:

I think she felt terrible guilt... how she'd been happy just to let things tick along and I think she realised that it was detrimental to her brother.

Knowing that the placement was time-limited, Matt worked closely with staff on a detailed care plan which defined specific goals. The staff then took on the day-to-day work with David, and Matt reviewed progress every three months. In many areas, David had to start from scratch. As well as communication, he had to learn the basics of money, going to the shops, getting on a bus, managing a home, as well as fundamental things like understanding the concept of time:

> *Time's meaningless really when you don't know what it is. What's ten minutes, what's a week?*

All of this took a lot of work by David and his support workers, but when, a couple of years later, a vacancy came up in an independent flat with support, Matt felt that David was ready to make the move. By now, he had many more strategies for communicating his wishes and, when he had been to see the flat, he immediately made his feelings very clear:

> *He must have understood what people were trying to indicate to him because he started writing down his name with the number of the flat and cutting out things from Argos catalogues like sofas and kettles. So, he really wanted to go. That was his way of saying 'yes I want that flat – that's got my name on it'.*

David's life is now very different from how it used to be. He knows many of his neighbours and has a circle of Deaf friends. It is still difficult for him to talk about his feelings and emotions as he does not have the words to describe them. But, he communicates more concrete concepts using a mixture of sign language, pictures, photos, words and symbols. He is able to use a calendar and tell the time so that he can keep appointments without having to be reminded. He now catches the bus on his own to the workshop and has started going to a fitness class at the sports centre, meeting a group of friends for a coffee afterwards. Staff at the housing scheme still support him with cooking, shopping, money management and communication and have helped him and some of his neighbours to go on holiday together. His self-confidence has grown and he now takes pride in his appearance and enjoys buying new clothes for himself. As David's independence has increased, Matt's involvement has decreased and he now just reviews David's support just once a year.

Discussion

This story amply demonstrates that social work with older people is about much more than law, policy and procedure. As in all the cases we have looked at, Matt was consciously working within the Mental Capacity Act 2005. His starting point was to assume that David had the capacity to make decisions about his future and to work with him on that basis. However, the motivation behind his work was an ethical one – a strong sense that David had been discriminated against in a way that had had a profoundly limiting impact on his life. David appeared content at home and did not seem to want anything to change. His family were not uncaring and he generally got on well with them. However, Matt recognised that David was not able to make choices about his life because he had no idea what could be different. A less committed social worker, or one who was not prepared (or not allowed) to spend as much time, might well have concluded that there was no need to intervene.

By contrast, Matt's work with David is an exemplary case study in rights-based social work and the benefits of positive risk-taking or 'risk-enablement'. At home, David's parents were very protective. Virtually all risks were avoided so that David was 'safe'. However, in order to have a more interesting and fulfilling life, he had to take risks when going out on his own, like negotiating roads or handling money. Part of Matt's work was to manage this process so that the potential dangers were weighed up against the potential benefits. Matt certainly was not cavalier in the way he did this and his approach was one of 'informed risk-taking' (O'Sullivan, 2009, p. 202). So, when David first started going to the supermarket to do his own shopping, it was agreed that his support staff would follow him at a distance to observe how he got on. Although he was able to buy things, he tended just to get chocolate and other treats rather than 'proper' food and, if he found he had bought more than he could carry, he would simply leave it behind in the shop. He was also very trusting and, rather than working out the money himself, would hand his purse over to the cashier, leaving himself very vulnerable. As a result, the support workers continued to support him with shopping and tried to work with him on ideas of personal safety. Even so, Matt felt this was a continuing area of risk:

> *That's still a worrying area for him. How do you ever explain to somebody like that that not everybody is good. That some people might want to hurt you. He has probably – I'm assuming – never had a sexual relationship and wouldn't understand about saying no, wouldn't understand about sexual health – he's missed all of that.*

Matt also went to great lengths to involve David in all the decisions that were being made. In his life up to that point, David had had virtually no autonomy. It was difficult for him to make decisions because he had very little experience of choice:

> *Always in my mind [I wanted] him to understand about the decisions that were being made so that he could be as involved as possible and consenting. 'Cos I think it's very easy with someone like him just to push him along. He could have ended up anywhere – in a completely inappropriate place. He wouldn't have known that he could say that he didn't want something. ... How can you decide if you want to go to the cinema or swimming if you've never been; [or about] food, never having had to make choices about what to have for dinner. And then suddenly you get to choose.*

Matt had to work out how best to support David to make decisions. It was not just a question of giving him information, because David, with so little experience and language, was not necessarily able to use it. Paradoxically, Matt's good judgement was in deciding not only what information to give him, but also what to withhold, so that the decisions that needed to be made were in terms that David could understand. Matt discussed this when describing the reviews he did with David:

> *What is really nice now with the review meetings, is that I try to work in a very person-centred way ... and the review [gives] him the opportunity to take the lead. Hopefully, he'll bring along something that he has prepared to tell me about how his year has been and things that he wants to carry on the same – things that he likes and things that he doesn't like, things that he wants to change. And that tends to work quite well. And if there are any wider service issues I would talk about that separately with staff as he wouldn't be included – it would be tokenistic to start talking about funding and personal budgets and things like that. If he wasn't happy about something, I would have to offer an alternative in a very concrete way. [Talking about] concepts and things for someone in the very early stages of learning a language is very difficult. ...*
>
> *I think bombarding people with too much information is irrelevant. That's where we, as social workers, have to use our judgement.*

All of this required Matt to know David very well – almost to start making some of his choices for him, so that they could be narrowed down to a point at which David could take part. There is a complex dynamic going on here between giving clear guidance and promoting choice – a sense in which Matt has to take control in order to give David control. So, for example, it was Matt who decided initially that a residential home would not be the right environment for David, even though his sister thought that it would be. Instead, he showed David the shared house and established that David would like to live there. It was Matt who actually decided to intervene at all, even though David was not obviously unhappy at home and, knowing nothing different, would probably have been reasonably content in residential care.

The outcomes of social work interventions are frequently mixed. Often the best we can achieve is to make a situation more manageable, or prevent it from getting worse. It is quite unusual for a social worker to be instrumental in such a complete and positive transformation of someone's life and Matt's pleasure in the outcome and pride and amazement at what David has achieved is palpable:

> *On bad days, when I think of the likes of him – that one case makes it all worthwhile really.*

18 Conclusion

A best practice approach

As we said in the Introduction, social workers often shy away from describing the work they do in positive terms. It may be that we are simply unwilling to 'blow our own trumpets', but the argument we have put forward in this book is that social work has developed a default position of negativity, a 'deficit culture', which has come to characterise much of what is said and written about it. At first sight, the notion of 'best practice' may appear to be a problematic one: there is something hard and definitive-sounding about the word 'best', which seems out of place in a profession that has taken critical reflection to its heart. However, in his book on social work theory, David Howe (2009) helpfully looks at the ways in which 'best' is used both to describe an objective, measurable outcome (the best score in a competition) and a subjective value (the best meal). He argues that, in social work, as in much of life, the judgements that we make involve both quantitative and qualitative evaluation – weighing up hard, factual evidence along with our own and others' experiences, moral values, feelings and relationships. The question social workers constantly have to ask themselves is 'What is the best course of action in this case?' (p. 201). This is an ordinary, not an exceptional kind of 'best' – the best that we can do with this person, at this time, within this set of circumstances. And of course, in most cases, the course of action depends primarily not on the social workers, but on the clients themselves.

In their critically reflective approach to their work, the social workers we interviewed were all too well aware of the elusiveness of a 'best' course of action: Nada questioned whether she had been too persuasive when Joan agreed to move into a care home, whilst Fiona questioned whether she had been persuasive enough when Ester decided against a placement. In the end, it is this very questioning which characterises good social work – arriving through empathetic listening, analysis and critical reflection at what seems to be the best course of action.

It is also worth repeating that the stories in this book do not provide a blueprint for practice. Instead, a 'best practice approach' should be understood as a way of engaging the reader in a debate about what it is that makes social work good. It is a 'bottom-up' approach, presenting the 'talking knowledge' (Gordon and Cooper, 2010, p. 246) of social workers as a way of stimulating discussion and learning. The purpose of this kind of detailed, situated analysis is precisely to provide an alternative (and a challenge) to the more idealised, prescriptive writing of many academic texts and policy documents, 'where practitioners are told what they *should* be doing, but never how, or considering even if it is possible' (Jones et al., 2008b, p. 289). The 'big story' of how people can best be helped and society transformed needs to be told. But, alongside it are thousands of small, detailed stories in which social workers have to scale these overarching narratives down to particular person's life, with all its ambiguities and contradictions.

The best social work and the best social workers

It may not be possible to look at a particular example of social work practice and call it categorically 'best' in a definitive sense of the word. However, it would be quite wrong to conclude that nothing can be said about the characteristics of the best social work, or about the qualities of the social workers who practice it. In fact, it is odd (if symptomatic of a 'deficit culture') that social work continues to find it so difficult to develop a strong identity, when there are so many themes that reoccur again and again in social work research and literature. Perhaps we have become so used to social work being contested from within and criticised from without, that we have lost sight of what we clearly can say about best practice. Maybe it is not as contested as we think.

In the stories presented in this book, we have seen how the best social workers have many attributes in common. Some of these will have been acquired through education and experience: others, although cultivated and honed, will be fundamentally intuitive or dispositional. The stories we have looked at show social workers who are knowledgeable, authoritative and pragmatic. They have a confident, internalised understanding of law and policy. They humanise managerial systems and make them effective, balancing the need for overall equity with a commitment to their particular clients. They focus on achievable solutions, building on people's strengths and remaining optimistic and hopeful. At the same time, they subject their work to intensive critical reflection and analysis. Whilst being respectful of the views of others they are also sceptical and prepared to be 'uncertain' as they negotiate ways forward with people who disagree with each other. They are committed to their clients' rights and habitually reflect on the power differentials that suffuse people's lives, scrutinising particularly closely their own position of influence and authority. They are attuned to the ways in which the structures of organised welfare perpetuate injustice and inequality and look for opportunities to challenge and change them. And they use their knowledge, critical reflection and ethical reasoning to make confident and defensible decisions.

But, perhaps what these stories illuminate above all is the compassion and commitment of the best social workers. They are professionally but unfailingly caring (and often simply kind), spending time getting to know their clients and trying to understand how they think their lives could change for the better. Their interest in the people they encounter is genuine, sometimes revealing a real delight in human variety, with all its attendant eccentricities and foibles. All of these are characteristics that have been tried and tested in social work, some of them over a considerable period of time. As David Howe puts it:

> ...when you read accounts of social work practice written 60, 80, 100 or more years ago...they feel and sound stubbornly familiar. This doesn't mean that new ideas aren't being incorporated into practice. Rather, these ideas get woven into the more densely textured fabric of the actuality of day-to-day practice, through rarely in a pure, unadulterated form. (2009, p. 193)

Looking to the future

We set out to write a positive book, a book that both celebrates and encourages readers to learn from best practice and communicates a justifiable (if unfamiliar) sense of pride in the profession. Sometimes this has not felt easy, faced with the shortcomings of an apparently ubiquitous managerial culture and the reluctance of policy-makers to acknowledge that real improvements need proper resourcing as well as 'choice' and 'flexibility'. But it has also been rewarding to do and we have found ourselves both inspired and encouraged by the practice we have heard about.

There is, however, a real value in positive thinking, beyond that of learning and celebration. Social work takes place within a political context which is constantly changing, subject to shifting ideologies and budgetary constraints and, as long as there is statutory welfare provision, it is highly likely that this will always be the case. At the time of writing, we are at the start of the biggest upheaval in adult social care in England since the 1990 NHS and Community Care Act. Personal Budgets are being introduced and, following the report by the Dilnot Commission (Dilnot et al., 2011), decisions will have to be made about how care for older people is funded. The Health and Social Care Act 2012 has made fundamental changes to health commissioning arrangements, placing an emphasis on close working between health and social care services. Adult care legislation is being revised and rationalised in a new Care and Support Bill which, amongst other things, will put local authorities' responsibility for Safeguarding Adults on a statutory footing. In amongst all this, fundamental issues are being debated. To what extent should the state be responsible? Why can't older people or their families arrange their own care? Who should pay and how much? And, inevitably, there are questions about the role of social workers and whether, in fact, older people need them all.

These are the debates in 2013 and, by the time you read this, they may have changed. But the point is that, whatever the debates are, it is difficult to imagine that any reforms in public policy will fundamentally change the need that many older people have for skilled, effective social work. The problems of people's lives are simply too intractable and their very human complexity cannot simply be 'organised' away by changes to a system. 'Older people' are, of course, not a homogeneous group. There are clearly many who, given money and good information, are able to make their own care arrangements: many people with enough savings choose to do this already. They need expert advice and practical support, which may be provided by social workers, but does not constitute social work itself. However, other older people have had histories and experiences that make their lives extremely difficult, whether or not they have the financial resources to pay for their care. Age is often accompanied by physical and mental ill-health and people who have always made their own decisions and plans can find they are no longer able to do so. There are increasing numbers of older people living at home with complex health problems and dementia, often looked after by carers who are themselves well into their retirement. And there is a heightened awareness of abuse and evolving and complex case law around mental capacity. So, despite the naysayers, it seems very likely that social work with older people will become more necessary, and more in the spotlight, than ever before.

However, in order to be part of any ongoing debates and to influence the decisions that are made, social workers must find their voice and, in the words of The College of Social Work's mission statement:

> ... develop a strong profession, confident about the unique contributions it makes to the individuals, families and communities it serves, with a clear sense of its identity, values, ethics and purpose. (TCSW, 2012)

A strong, articulate profession will be able to speak out about the kinds of situations in which social work skills most need to be supported and developed: situations in which there are stressful relationships or complex family dynamics, questions around mental capacity, disagreement and conflict, abuse, self-neglect or high levels of risk. And it will be able to use its wealth of knowledge and experience to inform policy and challenge any developments that are counterproductive, unrealistic or unfair.

Good social work already has a clear identity but it needs to find a voice. Talking and writing with conviction and clarity about the work that we do is surely a good place to start.

References

Adams, R. (2002) 'Developing Critical Practice in Social Work' in R. Adams, L. Dominelli and M. Payne (eds) *Critical Practice in Social Work*. Basingstoke: Palgrave Macmillan.

Adams, R. (2009) 'Encountering Complexity and Uncertainty' in R. Adams, L. Dominelli and M. Payne (eds) *Practicing Social Work in a Complex World*. 2nd edn. Basingstoke: Palgrave Macmillan.

Adams, R., Dominelli, L. and Payne, M. (2009) 'Developing Integrative Practice' in R. Adams, L. Dominelli and M. Payne (eds) *Practicing Social Work in a Complex World*. 2nd edn. Basingstoke: Palgrave Macmillan.

Adams, R., Dominelli, L., Payne, M. (eds) (2009) *Practising Social Work in a Complex World*. Basingstoke: Palgrave Macmillan.

Alzheimers Society (2010) *Factsheet: Communicating*. http://www.alzheimers.org.uk (home page)

Baginsky, M., Moriarty, J. et al (2010) 'Social Workers' Workload Survey: Messages from the Frontline – Findings from the 2009 Survey and Interviews with Senior Managers'. http://dera.ioe.ac.uk/ (homepage)

Banks, S. (2007) 'Between Equity and Empathy: Social Professions and the New Accountability' *Social Work and Society, 5, Festschrift Walter Lorenz*. http://www.socwork.net (home page)

Banks, S. (2008) 'Critical Commentary: Social Work Ethics', *British Journal of Social Work*, 38, 1238–1249.

Barrett, G. and Keeping C. (2005) 'The Processes Required for Effective Interprofessional Working' in G. Barrett, D. Sellman, and J. Thomas (eds), *Interprofessional Working in Health and Social Care: Professional Perspectives*. Basingstoke: Palgrave Macmillan

Bennett, T., Cattermole, M. and Sanderson, H. (2009) *Outcome Focused Reviews: A Practical Guide*. London: Department of Health.

Beresford, P. and Croft, S. (2004) 'Service Users and Practitioners Reunited: The Key Component for Social Work Reform', *British Journal of Social Work*, 34, 53–68.

Beresford, P., Croft, S. and Adshead, L. (2008) '"We don't see her as a social worker": A Service User Case Study of the Importance of the Social Worker's Relationship and Humanity', *British Journal of Social Work*, 38, 1388–1407.

Bornat, J. and Byetheway, B. (2010) 'Perceptions and Presentations of Living with Everyday Risk in Later Life', *British Journal of Social Work*, 40, 1118–1134.

Bowey, L. and McGlaughin, A. (2005) 'Adults with a Learning Disability Living with Elderly Carers Talk about Planning for the Future: Aspirations and Concerns', *British Journal of Social Work*, 35, 1377–1392.

Bowey, L. and McGlaughin, A. (2007) 'Older Carers of Adults with a Learning Disability Confront the Future: Issues and Preferences in Planning', *British Journal of Social Work*, 37, 39–54.

Brechin, A. (2000) 'Introducing Critical Practice' in A. Brechin, H. Brown and M. Eby (eds) *Critical Practice in Health and Social Care*. London: Sage.

Cameron, W.B. (1963) *Informal Sociology: a Casual Introduction to Sociological Thinking*. New York: Random House.

Carr, S. (2010) *Personalisation, Productivity and Efficiency*, SCIE. http://www.scie.org.uk (home page).

Charles, M. and Butler, S. (2004) 'Social Workers' Management of Organisational Change' in M. Lymbery and S. Butler (eds) *Social Work Ideals and Practice Realities*. Basingstoke: Palgrave Macmillan.

Clark, A. and Lynch, R. (2010) 'Older People' in S.J. Hothersall and M. Maas-Lowit (eds) *Need, Risk and Protection in Social Work Practice*. Exeter: Learning Matters.

Collins, S. (2008) 'Statutory Social Workers: Stress, Job Satisfaction, Coping, Social Support and Individual Differences', *British Journal of Social Work*, 38, 1173–1193.

Cook, G., Gerrish, K. and Clark, C. (2001) 'Decision Making in Teams: Issues Arising from Two UK Evaluations', *Journal of Interprofessional Care*, 15, 141–151.

Cooper, B. (2008) 'Best Practice in Social Work Interviewing: Processes of Negotiation and Assessment' in K. Jones, B. Cooper and H. Ferguson (eds) *Best Practice in Social Work: Critical Perspectives*. Basingstoke: Palgrave Macmillan.

Coulshed, V. (1991) *Social Work Practice: An Introduction*. Basingstoke: Palgrave/BASW.

Cree, V. and Wallace, S. (2009) 'Risk and Protection' in R. Adams, L. Dominelli, M. Payne (eds) *Practicing Social Work in a Complex World*. Basingstoke: Palgrave Macmillan.

Davis, A. and Garrett, M. (2004) 'Progressive Practice for Tough Times: Social Work, Poverty and Division in the Twenty-first Century' in M. Lymbery and S. Butler (eds) *Social Work Ideals and Practice Realities*. Basingstoke: Palgrave Macmillan.

de Boer, C. and Coady, N. (2007) 'Good Helping Relationships in Child Welfare: Learning from Success', *Child and Family Social Work*, 12, 32–42.

Dilnot, A., Warner, N. and Williams J. (2011) *Fairer Care Funding: The Report of the Commission on Funding of Care and Support*, Crown Copyright. http://www.dilnotcommission.dh.gov.uk (home page)

Douglass, H. (2005) 'The Development of Practice Theory in Adult Protection Intervention: Insights from a Recent Research Project' *The Journal of Adult Protection*, 7(1), 32–45.

Duffy, S. (2011) 'The Citizenship Theory of Social Justice: Exploring the Meaning of Personalisation for Social Workers', *Journal of Social Work Practice*, 24, 253–267.

Dwyer, S. (2005) 'Older People and Permanent Care: Whose Decision?', *British Journal of Social Work*, 35, 1081–1092.

Eby, M. (2000) 'The Challenges of Values and Ethics in Practice' in A. Brechin, H. Brown and M. Eby (eds) *Critical Practice in Health and Social Care*. London: Sage.

Equality and Human Rights Commission (2011), *Close to Home: An Inquiry into Older People and Human Rights in Home Care*. http://www.equalityhumanrights.com/homecareinquiry

Evans, T. and Harris, J. (2004) 'Street-Level Bureaucracy, Social Work and the (Exaggerated) Death of Discretion', *British Journal of Social Work*, 34, 871–895.

Ferguson, H. (2003) 'Outline of Critical Best Practice Perspective on Social Work and Social Care', *British Journal of Social Work*, 33, 1005–1024.

Ferguson, I. (2007) 'Increasing User Choice or Privatizing Risk? The Antinomies of Personalisation', *British Journal of Social Work*, 37, 387–403.

Ferguson, H. (2008) 'The Theory and Practice of Critical Best Practice in Social Work' in K. Jones, B. Cooper and H. Ferguson (eds) *Best Practice in Social Work: Critical Perspectives*. Basingstoke: Palgrave Macmillan.

Ferguson, H. (2010) 'Walks, Home Visits and Atmospheres: Risk and the Everyday Practices and Mobilities of Social Work and Child Protection', *British Journal of Social Work*, 40, 1100–1117.

Ferguson, I. and Woodward, R. (2009) *Radical Social Work in Practice: Making a Difference*. Bristol: The Policy Press.

Fook, J. (2002) *Social Work: Critical Theory and Practice*. London: Sage.

Frank, A. (2004) *The Renewal of Generosity*. Chicago: University of Chicago Press.

Frost, L. and Hoggett, P. (2008), 'Human Agency and Social Suffering', *Critical Social Policy*, 28(4), 438–460.

Gaylard, D. (2009) 'Assessing Adults' in A. Mantel (ed) *Social Work Skills with Adults*, Exeter: Learning Matters.

Glendinning, C., Clarke, S., Hare, P., Kotchetkova, I., Maddison, J. and Newbronner, L. (2006) *Outcomes-Focused Services for Older People*. London: Social Care Institute for Excellence.

Gordon, J. and Cooper, B. (2010) 'Talking Knowledge – Practising Knowledge: A Critical Best Practice Approach to How Social Workers Understand and Use Knowledge in Practice', *Practice: Social Work in Action*, 22(4), 245–257.

Gorman, H. (2000) 'Winning Hearts and Minds? – Emotional Labour and Learning for Care Management Work', *Journal of Social Work Practice*, 14(2), 149–158

Great Britain, Department for Constitutional Affairs (2006) *A Guide to the Human Rights Act 1998*. 3rd edn., DCA. www.justice.gov.uk (home page).

Great Britain, Department for Constitutional Affairs (2007) *Mental Capacity Act 2005 Code of Practice*. London: The Stationery Office.

Great Britain, Department of Health (2000), No Secrets: Guidance on Developing and Implementing Multi-Agency Policies and Procedures to Protect Vulnerable Adults from Abuse, Department of Health, www.dh.gov.uk/publications

Great Britain, Department of Health (2005), Independence, Wellbeing and Choice: Our Vision for the Future of Social Care in England, Department of Health, www.dh.gov.uk (homepage).

Great Britain, Department of Health (2007a) Putting People First: a Shared Vision and Commitment to the Transformation of Adult Social Care, Department of Health, www.dh.gov.uk/publications.

Great Britain, Department of Health (2007b) Independence, Choice and Risk: a Guide to Best Practice in Supported Decision Making, Department of Health, www.dh.gov.uk/publications

Great Britain, Department of Health (2009) Safeguarding Adults: Report on the Consultation on the Review of 'No Secrets', Department of Health, www.dh.gov.uk/publications

Great Britain, Department of Health (2010a) Prioritising Need in the Context of Putting People First: A Whole System Approach to Eligibility for Social Care, Department of Health, http://www.dh.gov.uk/publications

Great Britain, Department of Health (2010b) Fairer Contributions Guidance 2010: Calculating an Individual's Contribution to Their Personal Budget, Department of Health, http://www.dh.gov.uk/publications

Great Britain, Department of Health (2010c) *A Vision for Adult Social Care: Capable Communities and Active Citizens*, Department of Health, http://www.dh.gov.uk/publications

Great Britain, Department of Health (2010d) *Building the National Care Service.* London: Department of Health.

Great Britain, Department of Health (2011) *The 2011/2012 Adult Social Care Outcomes Framework*, Department of Health, http://www.dh.gov.uk/publications

Great Britain, Department of Health (2012a) *Caring for Our Future.* London: TSO.

Great Britain, Department of Health (2012b) Fairer Charging Policies for Home Care and Other Non-Residential Social Services: Guidance for Councils with Social Services Responsibilities, Department of Health, www.dh.gov.uk (homepage)

Great Britain, Ministry of Justice (2008) *Mental Capacity Act 2005 Deprivation of Liberty Safeguards,* Ministry of Justice, www. dh.gov.uk/publications

Gregson, M. and Holloway, M. (2005) 'Language and the Shaping of Social Work', *British Journal of Social Work,* 35(1), 37–53.

Grenier, A. (2006) 'The Distinction Between Being and Feeling Frail: Exploring Emotional Experiences in Health and Social Care', *Journal of Social Work Practice,* 20(3), 299–313.

Hanley, P. (2009) 'Communication Skills in Social Work' in R. Adams, L. Dominelli and M. Payne (eds) *Social Work: Themes, Issues and Critical Debates,* 3rd ed. Basingstoke: Palgrave Macmillan.

Harrop, A. (2011), *Care in Crisis: Causes and Solutions,* Age UK. http://www.ageuk.org.uk/professional-resources

Health & Care Professionals Council (2012) Standards of Proficiency for Social Workers in England. www.hcpc-uk.org

Healy, K. (2005) *Social Work Theories in Context: Creating Frameworks for Practice.* Basingstoke: Palgrave Macmillan.

Hoggett, P. (2001) 'Agency, Rationality and Social Policy', *Journal of Social Policy,* 30(1), 37–56.

Howe, D. (1993) *On Being a Client: Understanding the Process of Counselling and Psychotherapy.* London: Sage.

Howe, D. (1994) 'Modernity, Postmodernity and Social Work', *British Journal of Social Work,* 25, 513–532.

Howe, D. (2008) *The Emotionally Intelligent Social Worker.* Basingstoke: Palgrave Macmillan.

Howe, D. (2009) *A Brief Introduction to Social Work Theory.* Basingstoke: Palgrave Macmillan.

Hugman, R. (2000) 'Older People and Their Families: Rethinking the Social Work Task', *Australian Social Work,* 53(1), 3–8.

Hugman, R. (2003) 'Professional Values and Ethics in Social Work: Reconsidering Postmodernism', *British Journal of Social Work,* 33, 1025–1041.

Hughes, M. and Wearing, M. (2007) *Organisations and Management in Social Work.* London: Sage.

James, O. (2008) *Contented Dementia.* Chatham: Vermilion Ebury Publishing.

Jones, K., Cooper, B. and Ferguson, H. (2008a) 'Introducing Critical Best Practice in Social Work' in K. Jones, B. Cooper and H. Ferguson (eds) *Best Practice in Social Work: Critical Perspectives.* Basingstoke: Palgrave Macmillan.

Jones, K., Cooper, B. and Ferguson, H. (2008b) 'Concluding Reflections on the Nature and Future of Critical Best Practice' in K. Jones, B. Cooper, and H. Ferguson (eds) *Best Practice in Social Work: Critical Perspectives.* Basingstoke: Palgrave Macmillan.

Jones, K. and Powell, I. (2008) 'Situating Person and Place: Best Practice in Dementia Care' in K. Jones, B. Cooper and H. Ferguson (eds) *Best Practice in Social Work: Critical Perspectives.* Basingstoke: Palgrave Macmillan.

Jones, K. and Spreadbury, K. (2008) 'Best Practice in Adult Protection: Safety, Choice and Inclusion' in K. Jones, B. Cooper and H. Ferguson (eds) *Best Practice in Social Work: Critical Perspectives.* Basingstoke: Palgrave Macmillan.

Jordan, B. (2001) 'Tough Love: Social Work, Social Exclusion and the Third Way', *British Journal of Social Work*, 31(4), 527–546.

Kadushin, A. (1990) *The Social Work Interview. A Guide for Human Service Professionals*, 3rd edn. New York: Columbia University Press.

Kahneman, D. (2011) *Thinking, Fast and Slow*. London: Penguin.

Kemshall, H. (2002) *Risk, Social Policy and Welfare*. Buckingham: Open University Press.

Kitwood, T. (1997) 'The Experience of Dementia', *Aging and Mental Health*, 1(1), 13–22.

Kroll, B. (2010) 'Only Connect... Building Relationships with Hard-to-Reach People: Establishing Rapport with Drug-misusing Parents and their Children' in G. Ruch, D. Turney and A. Ward (eds) *Relationship-Based Social Work: Getting to the Heart of Practice*. London: Jessica Kingsley.

Lindsay, P. (2008) 'Sunrise, Sunset – the Transitions Faced by the Parents of Adults with Learning Disabilities', *Advances in Mental Health and Learning Disabilities*, 2(3), 13–17.

Lloyd, L. (2003) 'Caring Relationships: Looking beyond Welfare Categories of 'Carers' and 'Service Users' in S. Stalker (ed.) *Reconceptualising Work with 'Carers'*. London: Jessica Kingsley.

Lloyd, L. (2006) 'A Caring Profession? The Ethics of Care and Social Work with Older People', *British Journal of Social Work*, 36, 1171–1185.

Loxley, A. (1997) *Collaboration in Health and Welfare: Working with Difference*. London: Jessica Kingsley Publishers.

Lymbery, M. (2004) 'Managerialism and Care Management Practice with Older People' in M. Lymbery and S. Butler (eds) *Social Work Ideals and Practice Realities*. Basingstoke: Palgrave Macmillan.

Lymbery. M. and Butler, S. (2004) 'Social Work Ideals and Practice Realities: An Introduction' in M. Lymbery and S. Butler (eds) *Social Work Ideals and Practice Realities*. Basingstoke: Palgrave Macmillan.

Lymbery, M. (2005) *Social Work with Older People*. London: Sage.

Lymbery, M. (2006) 'United We Stand? Partnership Working in Health and Social Care and the Role of Social Work in Services for Older People', *British Journal of Social Work*, 36, 1119 1134.

Lymbery, M. and Postle, K. (2010) 'Social Work in the Context of Adult Social Care in England and the Resultant Implications for Social Work Education', *British Journal of Social Work*, 40, 2502–2522.

McDonald, A. (2010) *Need, Risk and Protection in Social Work*. Bristol: The Policy Press.

Macdonald, G. and Macdonald, K., 'Safeguarding: A Case for Intelligent Risk Management', *British Journal of Social Work*, 40, 1174–1191.

Manthorpe, J. et al. (2008) 'There Are Wonderful Social Workers but It's a Lottery: Older People's Views about Social Workers', *British Journal of Social Work*, 38, 1132–1150.

Mantell, A. and Clark, A. (2011) 'Making Choices: The Mental Capacity Act 2005' in T. Scragg and A. Mantel (eds) *Safeguarding Adults in Social Work*, 2nd edn. Exeter: Learning Matters.

McBeath, G. and Webb, S. (2002) 'Virtue Ethics and Social Work: Being Lucky, Realistic and not Doing One's Duty', *British Journal of Social Work*, 32, 1015–1036.

Melanie Henwood Associates (2011) Journeys without Maps: The Decisions and Destinations of People Who Self Fund. Putting People First Consortium.

Morrison, T. (2007) 'Emotional Intelligence, Emotion and Social Work: Contexts, Characteristics, Complications and Contribution', *British Journal of Social Work*, 37, 245–263.

Munro, E. (2002) *Effective Child Protection*. London: Sage.

Munro, E. (2011) The Munro Review of Child Protection: Final Report – A Child Centred System, www. education.gov.uk (home page)

Nuffield Foundation on Bioethics (2009) *Dementia: Ethical Issues.* Cambridge: Nuffield Foundation.

O'Hagan, M. (2000) 'Two Accounts of Mental Distress' in J. Read and J. Reynolds (eds) *Speaking Our Minds.* Basingstoke: Palgrave Macmillan.

O'Sullivan, T. (2009) 'Managing Risk and Decision-Making' in R. Adams, L. Dominelli and M. Payne (eds) *Practicing Social Work in a Complex World.* Basingstoke: Palgrave Macmillan.

O'Sullivan, T. (2011) *Decision Making in Social Work,* 2nd edn. Basingstoke: Palgrave Macmillan.

Osmond, J. and O'Connor, I. (2004) 'Formalising the Unformalised: Practitioners' Communication of Knowledge in Practice', *British Journal of Social Work,* 34, 677–692.

Parker, G. and Clarke, H. (2002). 'Making the Ends Meet: Do Carers and Disabled People have a Common Agenda?' *Policy and Politics,* 30(3), 347–359.

Parton, N. and O'Byrne, P. (2000) 'What Do We Mean by Constructive Social Work?' in N. Parton and P. O'Byrne (eds), *Constructive Social Work:Towards a New Practice.* London: Macmillan.

Parton, N. (2003) 'Rethinking *Professional* Practice: The Contributions of Social Constructionism and the Feminist 'Ethics of Care', *British Journal of Social Work,* 33, 1–16.

Payne, M. (2012) *Citizenship Social Work with Older People.* Bristol: Policy Press.

Postle, K. (2002) 'Working "Between the Idea and the Reality": Ambiguities and Tensions in Care Managers' Work', *British Journal of Social Work,* 32(3), 335–351.

Pritchard, J. (2001) 'Neglect: Not Grasping the Nettle and Hiding behind Choice' in J. Pritchard (ed.) *Good Practice with Vulnerable Adults.* London: Jessica Kingsley.

Ray, M., Bernard, M. and Phillips, J. (2009) *Critical Issues in Social Work with Older People.* Basingstoke: Palgrave Macmillan.

Saleeby, D. (ed) (2006) *The Strengths Perspective in Social Work Practice,* 4th edn. Boston: Pearson.

Sandel, M.J. (2010) *Justice: What's the Right Thing to Do?* London: Penguin.

Sayce, L. (2009) 'Rights, Risks and Anti-Discrimination Work in Mental Health' in R. Adams, L. Dominelli, M. Payne (eds) *Practicing Social Work in a Complex World.* Basingstoke: Palgrave Macmillan.

Schön, D. (1987) *Educating the Reflective Practitioner.* San Francisco: Jossey Bass.

Schön, D. (1993) *The Reflective Practitioner.* Aldershot: Arena.

Seddon, J. (2008) *Systems Thinking in the Public Sector: The Failure of the Reform Regime ... and a Manifesto for a Better Way.* Axminster: Triarchy Press.

Sen, A. (2009) *The Idea of Justice.* London: Penguin.

Senior, B. and Loades, E. (2008) 'Best Practice as Skilled Organisational Work' in K. Jones, B. Cooper and H. Ferguson (eds) *Best Practice in Social Work: Critical Perspectives.* Basingstoke: Palgrave Macmillan.

Sennett, R. (2003) *Respect.* London: Penguin.

Sheldon, B. and Maconald, G. (2009) *A Textbook of Social Work,* 4th edn. Abingdon: Routledge.

Shulman, L. (1999) The Skills of Helping Individuals, Families, Groups and Communities. Itasca, IL: Peacock.

Smethurst, C. (2011) 'Working with Risk' in T. Scragg and A. Mantel (eds) *Safeguarding Adults in Social Work,* 2nd edn. Exeter: Learning Matters.

Social Care Institute for Excellence (2005) Research Briefing 12: Involving Individual Older Patients and Their Carers in the Discharge Process from Acute to Community Care: Implications for Immediate Care. http://www.scie.org.uk (home page)

Social Care Institute for Excellence (2010), Enabling Risk, Ensuring Safety: Self-directed Support and Personal Budgets, www.scie.org.uk (home page)

Social Work Task Force (2009) Final Report of the Social Work Task Force: Building a Safe and Confident Future, http://publications.dcsf.gov.uk

Stevenson, O. (1971), 'Knowledge for Social Work', British Journal of Social Work, 1(2), 225–237.

Stevenson, O. (2004) 'The Future of Social Work' in M. Lymbery and S. Butler (eds.) Social Work Ideals and Practice Realities. Basingstoke: Palgrave Macmillan.

Tanner, D. and Harris, J. (2008) Working with Older People. Abingdon: Routledge.

Taylor, B. and Donnelly, M. (2006) 'Professional Perspectives on Decision Making about the Long-Term Care of Older People', British Journal of Social Work, 36, 807–826.

Taylor, C. and White, S. (2006), 'Knowledge and Reasoning in Social Work: Educating for Humane Judgement', British Journal of Social Work, 36, 937–954.

The College of Social Work (2012), Mission Statement. http://www.collegeofsocialwork.org

The College of Social Work (2013), Professional Capabilities Framework. http://www.collegeofsocialwork.org

Thompson, N. (2000) Understanding Social Work: Preparing for Practice. Basingstoke: Palgrave Macmillan

Thompson, N. (2006) Anti-discriminatory Practice. Basingstoke: Palgrave Macmillan.

Trevithick, P. (2003) 'Effective Relationship-based Practice: A Theoretical Exploration', Journal of Social Work Practice, 17(2), 163–176.

Trevithick, P. (2005) Social Work Skills: A Practice Handbook. Buckingham: Open University Press.

Tulloch, J. and Lupton, D. (2003) Risk in Everyday Life. London: Sage.

Twigg, J. and Atkin, K. (1994) Carers Perceived: Policy and Practice in Informal Care. Buckingham: Open University.

Webb, S. (2006), Social Work in a Risk Society. Basingstoke: Palgrave Macmillan.

Weick, A. (2000) 'Hidden Voices', Social Work, 45, 5.

Weick, A, Rapp, C., Sullivan, W.P. and Kisthardt, W. (1989) 'A Strengths Perspective for Social Work Practice', Social Work, 34(4), 350–354.

Weingarten, K. (1997) 'Foreword' in C. White and J. Hales (eds) The Personal Is the Professional: Therapists reflect on their Families, Lives and Work. Adelaide: Dulwich Centre Publications.

Wilson, A. and Beresford, P. (2000) 'Anti-oppressive Practice: Emancipation or Appropriation', British Journal of Social Work, 30(5), 553–573.

Wilson, K., Ruch, G., Lymbery, M. and Cooper, A. (2011) Social Work Practice: An introduction to Contemporary Practice. Harlow: Pearson Education.

Witkin, S. (2000), 'Writing Social Work', Social Work, 45(5), 389–394.

Wilder Craig, R. (2007) 'A Day in the Life of a Hospital Social Worker: Presenting Our Role Through the Personal Narrative', Qualitative Social Work, 6, 431–446.

Yelloly, M. and Henkel, M. (eds) (1995) Learning and Teaching in Social Work: Towards Reflective Practice. London: Jessica Kingsley.

Index